Hospital-acquired Infection
Causes and Control

In consequence of my conviction I must affirm that only God knows the number of patients who went prematurely to their graves because of me. I have examined corpses to an extent equalled by few other obstetricians. If I say this also of another physician, my intention is only to bring to consciousness a truth that, to humanity's great misfortune, has remained unknown through so many centuries. No matter how painful and oppressive such a recognition may be, the remedy does not lie in suppression. If the misfortune is not to persist forever, then this truth must be made known to everyone concerned.

Ignacz Semmelweis, The Etiology, Concept, and Prophylaxis of Childbed Fever

Hospital-acquired Infection

Causes and Control

ZSOLT FILETOTH, MD, MSc

Head of Clinical Epidemiology Unit of the
National Institute of Traumatology, Budapest, Hungary

and

Consultant in Infectious Disease and Epidemiology,
National Institute of Neurosurgery, Budapest, Hungary

W
WHURR PUBLISHERS
LONDON AND PHILADELPHIA

© 2003 Whurr Publishers Ltd
First published 2003
by Whurr Publishers Ltd
19b Compton Terrace, London N1 2UN England and
325 Chestnut Street, Philadelphia PA 19106 USA

British Library Cataloguing in Publication Data

A catalogue record for this book is available from the British Library.

ISBN: 1 86156 344 2

Printed and bound in the UK by Athenaeum Press Ltd,
Gateshead, Tyne & Wear.

Contents

The author

Zsolt Filetoth was born in 1961 and grew up in Hungary. In 1979, after finishing high school in Budapest, he entered medical school in St Petersburg, Russia, where he graduated as an MD in 1985.

In 1985 he became a resident and clinical fellow in infectious disease and received training in hospital hygiene in Hungary. He organized the first course in Hungary in hospital-acquired infection for senior nurses and operating room nurses, which was recognized by the Postgraduate School for Nurses of Hungary. In 1992 and 1993 he studied basic epidemiology in the USA at the Centers for Disease Control and Prevention, Atlanta, Georgia, completing courses in Hospital Epidemiology and International Epidemic Intelligence Services.

In 1995 he studied at the Public Health Laboratory Service, London, and received individual training in hospital infection control at the Middlesex Hospital. In 1998 he was awarded an MSc degree by the University of London and the Diploma in Communicable Disease Epidemiology by the London School of Hygiene and Tropical Medicine.

Since 1994 he has been head of the Clinical Epidemiology Department of the National Institute of Traumatology, Budapest, Hungary. In 1999 he was appointed as a consultant in infectious disease and epidemiology at the National Institute of Neurosurgery, Budapest, Hungary.

Professionally, he is interested in the epidemiology of infectious diseases, especially in the surveillance of nosocomial infections, and in antibiotic policy. He is practice oriented, collaborating in molecular epidemiology at the Institute of Medical Microbiology of the Semmelweis University of Budapest, Hungary. He is an invited lecturer in communicable disease epidemiology at medical schools throughout Hungary, and has presented more than 40 lectures in hospital infection control.

Acknowledgements

I should like to express my thanks to people who contributed to my professional development, to Professor Philip S. Brachmann at Emory University, Atlanta, to Barry Cookson at the Public Health Laboratory Service, London, to Donna Dryer at Parkland Memorial Hospital, Dallas, to all my teachers at the Centers for Disease Control and Prevention, Atlanta, and the London School of Hygiene and Tropical Medicine.

Some chapters of this book contain data collected by clinical epidemiological assistants: Fügedi Albert, Ringbauer Zsuzsanna, Ruszin Aniko, Jakab Zsuzsanna and Zsupos Edit. Many thanks for their contributions.

I really appreciate the help of David Stevens, Michael Howell, Simon Andrea, Kleerné Klement Zsuzsanna, and librarians Almásyné Kovács Éva and Maderspack Károlyné in the technical preparation of the manuscript.

Finally I should like to express my gratitude to Tamásné Nagy Edit dr, who was my English language teacher.

Zsolt Filetoth

Preface

Hospital-acquired infection (HAI) is a complication of health care which affects on average 10% of patients admitted to hospitals worldwide. Such infections have serious public health implications by changing the quality of life of patients, and sometimes causing disability or even death. Moreover, the economic impact of HAI includes not only the cost of the extra time spent in hospital but also the increased cost to society due to lost working time, which also has financial implications for the patient and his/her family. It has been estimated that in the UK alone the annual cost of HAI is about £2 billion.

Infection control in hospital is an essential component of quality control in countries with high-quality healthcare. It began in the nineteenth century with the work of Florence Nightingale and Ignacz Semmelweis, who first recognized the importance of HAI. Today, the sickest patients admitted to hospital are the most susceptible to acquiring HAI, and the more invasive diagnostic and therapeutic procedures that they have to undergo increase the risk of opening the gates to further invasion of germs.

Medical staff must play a key role in the control of HAI because many of the procedures they undertake can lead to the development of HAI and to the transmission of nosocomial germs among patients. Their active participation is also important for self-defence, as they themselves can become infected during the care of infected patients.

The purpose of this book is to provide nurses and junior doctors with an understanding of the basics of infection control by explaining the methods employed and their purpose. It is based on lectures presented by the author at training courses for nurses and doctors, and gives simple, understandable and essential information that is vital knowledge for medical staff in hospitals. It is intended for both graduate and postgraduate levels.

Introduction

Hospital acquired infection (HAI) was first described in the nineteenth century. The antibiotic era, which began in 1929 with the discovery of penicillin by Fleming, has contributed much to the successful therapy of many infections. Antibiotics are used for both prophylactic and therapeutic purposes but they alone are not able to control HAI. Eradication of HAI is still beyond the scope of medicine, despite its rapid development. Today's medicine is more invasive, which increases the risk of the development of HAI by providing more opportunities for the invasion of germs. Additionally, the proportion of the sickest, immuno-compromised patients has been increasing in hospitals, and these are at greater risk of acquiring infections. Many HAIs have been described, and their distribution varies widely. However, the most ubiquitous are: surgical wound infection, pneumonia, urinary tract infection, bloodstream infection, device-associated infections and decubitus, which are explained by the universal occurrence of those risk factors influencing these most common types of HAI.

Infections in hospitals are dynamic: patients, staff and visitors can import any kind of infection into hospital, and they can also acquire infections within hospital and carry infectious agents to other hospitals or into the community. The term 'nosocomial infection' is usually restricted to the infections that patients acquire in hospital, but has importance in occupational medicine as well. The development of infections follows certain well-defined rules, the understanding of which is important for prevention. The same rules apply to both HAI and infections acquired in the community. In addition, HAI have some specificities as they are mainly associated with invasive medical procedures.

This book is intended to provide a basic introduction to the subject. It summarizes the main topics that are important to understanding the general principles of the development of infections, which in turn is essential for the effective control of HAI. It is based on lectures presented by the author at seminars for the training of nurses and junior doctors. The chapters follow a progressive sequence. However, the different sections can be read independently to meet the individual needs of the reader looking for specific information. First, the causes and risk factors of HAI that determine the diversity of HAI are described. Microbiological diagnosis is discussed, which is essential to understand the importance of the diagnosis of infections. Special emphasis is given to the infection process and the transmission of infection agents as the fundamental basis of infection control. Characteristics of HAI are given to highlight their specific nature, which distinguishes them from infections in the community. All essential aspects of the prevention of HAI are discussed in order to apply them for successful infection control. Finally, the basic principles of the organization of modern infection control are given, setting out the minimum of quality control of health care in hospitals. Relevant updated references are given for further reading.

CHAPTER 1

Causes and determinants of hospital-acquired infection

Concept of causality

That the search for causes of disease has always been central to human inquiry since the time of ancient cultures is confirmed by the written records of those cultures. The concept of causality is the focus of all research into disease by observing that one event precedes another, and if this pattern is repeated, then the preceding event can be taken as the cause of the later one. The word 'cause' comes from Latin *causa* = cause, which means: 'Something that brings about a change; that which produces an effect' (Churchill's, 1989, p. 312).

Theory of causal pie

The theory of 'causal pie' has been developed in disease research to explain the multi-causal mechanism of the development of disease by using the analogy of a pie containing several slices called the 'essential causes', which are needed for a disease to develop (Rothman, 1976). The whole pie is regarded as 'sufficient causa' of a disease, i.e. a disease develops if all essential causa are present at the same time.

Causal pie assumes the multi-factorial nature of disease, which is generally accepted for infectious diseases, where micro-organisms are the essential causa of such health events. Lack of immunity of the host is the next essential slice of the pie, which is completed by the presence of a micro-organism leading to the 'sufficient causa' together.

Causality is a wider term than *aetiology*, which is usually taken to be the *main* or specific causa of a disease. The term 'aetiology' is of Greek origin: *aitia* = cause + *log(os)* a telling (Churchill's, 1989, p. 654).

Different patterns of the same disease are represented by different pies that contain the same main specific causes of the disease necessary to initiate the pathological process. However, the same causa may contribute to different diseases. For example, *Staphylococcus aureus* may cause skin infections (folliculitis, impetigo), sepsis, food poisoning or other diseases. And, for example, food poisoning may be caused by various microbes, such as *Salmonella, Clostridium botulinum* or *Bacillus subtilis* with different patterns (pies) of development.

Risk factors of health-related events

The term 'risk factor' has been developed in disease research in order to find determinants that influence the occurrence of a health-related event in a population. Risk factor: 'An aspect of personal behaviour or life-style, an environmental exposure, or an inborn or inherited characteristic, which on the basis of epidemiological evidence is known to be associated with health related condition(s) considered important to prevent' (Last, 1995, p. 148). In other words, 'risk factor' is a 'determinant', but not necessarily a causal factor. However, the presence of risk factors in a population should be taken into account because any change in their occurrence will change the occurrence of a health-related event with which they are associated.

Risk factors of infections and non-infectious diseases can be classified into four distinguishable groups according to their source and possible influence (see Figure 1.1).

Endogenous risk factors are those that originate in a patient in whom a disease develops, and such factors contribute to an increased risk of development of the disease of interest.

Exogenous risk factors are those factors originating from a source external to the patient in whom the disease occurs; such factors are often called 'environmental'.

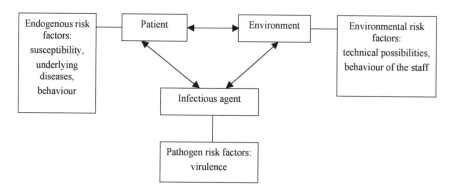

Figure 1.1. Risk factors of nosocomial infections.

Objective risk factors are mainly independent of humans, and are deter-mined mainly by nature.

Subjective risk factors depend on human decisions and interventions based on human behaviour.

Examples are:

- Endogenous objective risk factors – underlie diseases in a patient, and contribute to an increased susceptibility to infections that are the most important in the development of HAI.
- Endogenous subjective risk factors – behaviour, co-operation of a patient (psychiatric cases, conscious negligence) – also influence the occurrence of HAI at the individual level.
- Exogenous objective risk factors – the structure and technical capability of a health care system, and the development of medicine in general, to prevent and influence the occurrence of diseases, which also applies to HAI.
- Exogenous subjective risk factors – behaviour, attitudes and knowledge of those humans who influence the development of health-related events in *other* persons. Hospital staff play an important role in HAI – their conscious behaviour may prevent or promote the occurrence of HAI in patients. However, their behaviour plays an important role in self-defence because the HAIs have occupational importance.

Micro-organisms as essential causes of infectious diseases

In the development of research methods for observing our physical surroundings, the first important event occurred in the seventeenth century when Lewenhook constructed the first microscope from lenses, increasing the resolution capacity of our eyes and making visible those structures that are smaller than 0.1 millimetre. However, until the end of the nineteenth century the organisms seen under the Lewenhook microscope were not regarded as the causes of diseases. The work of Louis Pasteur and Robert Koch demonstrated that organisms seen by means of the microscope (called micro-organisms) may cause diseases (known as the aetiology of such diseases).

In the nineteenth century microbiology was born as an independent science and since then it has been searching for undiscovered micro-organisms, classifying and characterizing them according to their different attrib-utes. Recognition of the transmission of micro-organisms from one host to another as the cause of the same disease led to the adoption of the term *infectious disease*, defining micro-organisms as the main cause of this group of diseases. The word 'infection' comes from the Latin, *infectio* = to dip in, to dye (*in* = into + *facere* = to make, to treat) (Churchill's, 1989, p. 939). Since then, more and more diseases – those thought to be non-infectious – have been found to be infections caused by microbes.

General classification of micro-organisms

Classification of micro-organisms used to be based on their phenotype characteristics, i.e. their external features:

- morphological signs
- biochemical features
- life cycle.

Micro-organisms sharing the same morphological and life cycle features are grouped into the main classes listed below, dividing the microbiology into different sub-sciences:

- prions
- viruses
- chlamydiae
- rickettsiae
- mycoplasmas
- bacteria
- fungi
- protozoa
- helminths
- arthropods.

The main classes of microbes are divided into families, subfamilies and genera, which consist of the species of micro-organisms sharing the same genetic sequence, or are very close to each other according to other characteristics. Owing to the rapid development of molecular biology through the use of methods of genetic engineering there is an ongoing refinement of the classification of the families of micro-organisms according to their genetic substance, replacing the 'phenotype classification' (Bruckner et al., 1999; Fauquet and Pringle, 1999; Garcia, 1999; Jousimies-Somer and Summanen, 1999; McGinnis et al., 1999; Miller, 1999b).

Mutation is the term used if the offspring differs from the parent in genetic content, due to the loss of unstable genes and nucleic acids, or the construction of new genes, or the acquisition of new genes from other species. Mutations result in phylogenetic diversity of the species and if such genetic changes are minor different subtypes (called strains) of the same species appear and circulate in the environment.

Taxonomy of all micro-organisms relies on phylogenetic diversity showing hierarchical distribution: class – family – subfamily – genera – type – subtype (variant) – strain. The name of a micro-organism – except prions and viruses – consists of two parts. The first shows the *genus* to which the particular micro-organism belongs and the second part names the *type* (*species*). For example, *Staphylococcus aureus* belongs to the genus *Staphylococcus*, which has other species such as *Staphylococcus epidermidis*, *Staphylococcus saprophyticus*, etc. Subtypes, or variants and strains, have the same common species name with the addition of the subtype characteristic; for example, extended spectrum beta lactamase (ESBL) producing *Klebsiella pneumoniae* (ESBL-KP), or methicillin-resistant *Staphylococcus aureus* (MRSA).

Historically, the term 'parasite' was used for protozoa, helminths and arthropods, and this terminology has remained. Parasitism was earlier attributed to only these three groups. However, this is not correct because parasitic association also occurs with other groups of microbes (see Chapter 2). Species of these three groups differ from other microbes in that they have a complex life cycle containing different morphological stages. They may have sexual and asexual forms, and replicate by direct (in one host) or indirect (in definitive and intermediate hosts) means through consecutive phases.

Theoretically, each species of the above-mentioned group may cause HAI if the circumstances are appropriate: a human or inanimate source and successful transmission within the hospital. However, the frequency of microbes causing HAI is distributed unequally, which explains their unequal occurrence and other characteristics such as susceptibility, transmission and risk factors (see Chapters 3, 4 and 6).

Prions

Prions are the most recently discovered infectious agents. They used to be taken as viruses (Bobowick et al., 1973). A prion is a protein that has a regulatory function, influencing the function of host cells. Each host has its own prions, and among them there are many of that do not cause any disorder. However, for several unknown reasons prions may become infective and cause disease that is due to structural changes of the protein. Such infectious diseases are usually specific and each prion affects only its own host:

- Creutzfeldt-Jakob disease – human
- kuru – human
- scrapie – sheep and goats
- bovine spongiform encephalopathy (BSE).

Creutzfeldt-Jakob disease has been found in hospital settings and is accepted as HAI caused by the prion being transmitted by transfusion and blood contaminants (Gajdusek et al., 1977). The prion of Creutzfeld-Jakob disease (CJD) affects the central nervous system causing psychiatric illness, which explains the most common occurrence of this disease in psychiatry (Bobowick et al., 1973). Owing to its relatively long incubation period (15–20 years) older people suffer from this illness. Kuru has occurred among cannibals in tropical countries of Africa and Asia and is transmitted by eating the brains of victims.

Since the 1990s, modified Creutzfeldt-Jakob disease has appeared among young people possibly infected from 'mad cows' at farms or by digesting the infected meat and other products (e.g. milk) of such animals. 'Mad cow disease' is caused by the prion of scrapie, which is originally a spongiform disease of sheep. The disease appeared among cows as a result of human intervention, as the cadavers of sheep had been used to feed cows since the 1980s. This serious intervention is unnatural as cows eat grass and they never eat sheep alive or dead! So far the modified variant of Creutzfeldt-Jakob disease (vCJD) has occurred only in the United Kingdom (Brown et al., 2001). Although there is not enough evidence of the possible transmission of this modified prion in a health care setting, logically it may occur in the same way as the original type of CJD.

Prions are extremely resistant in the environment, surviving in boiled or roast meat up to 350°C, and the meat remains infective via the digestive system. Prions survive routine sterilization methods by heat or chemical disinfection used in health care settings, and their resistance against radiation is also substantial (Gibbs et al., 1978; Brown et al., 2001).

Currently the diagnosis of CJD and vCJD is based on clinical symptoms and histopathological changes in the brain. To date no standardized serological or other method for early diagnosis or screening has been developed. No test is so far available for checking blood donors and blood products.

Viruses

Viruses are the most frequent causes of infection after bacteria and fungi, both in the community and in hospitals. They are smaller than other organisms, with a size of 10 to 300 nm. Their structure consists of a core genetic substance and a protein coat that may contain lipid and other molecules. The genetic substance can be either DNA or RNA. Viruses can live and multiply only in the living cells of hosts (bacteria, plants, animals and humans). Viruses living in the cells of bacteria are called phages or bacteriophages.

Viruses do not have metabolic activity outside the host cells. The virus affecting the host cells forces the cells to do what is coded in the virus's genes, like a tape-machine plays the contents of a cassette. Viral infections can result in several characteristic clinical pictures:

- Replication of viruses in the cells occurs, producing free virions that leave the host cells by lysis or in some other way. The type of organ and the number of dead host cells determine the clinical picture and the severity of illness. This outcome serves to spread the virus into the environment.
- The virus gene integrates into the host's chromosome, leading to the carrier stage with the survival of both the host's cells and virus genome.
- The virus changes the surface antigen features of the host's cells leading to chronic and autoimmune disorders.
- There is benign or malignant growth of cells infected by the virus.

Viruses have been classified in various ways for different purposes:

- taxonomic
- Boston system
- clinical
- epidemiological.

Taxonomic classification is based on gene type (DNA or RNA) and on the main morphological characteristics (types of protein coat and other characteristics). It is important mainly for microbiologist-virologists. Viruses belonging to the same taxonomic group may have different epidemiological features and different clinical outcomes (see Table 1.1). There are no specific rules in the naming of viruses – their name may reflect the main disease (e.g. hepatitis viruses causing mainly inflammation of the liver), or the place

Table 1.1. Medically important viruses with possible acquisition in hospitals

Family	Subfamily	Genus	Species	Genome type	Disease	Other characteristics	HAI
Adenoviridae		Mastadenovirus	Human adenovirus A – F (HadV)	DS DNA	acute haemorrhagic syndrome: keratoconjunctivitis epidemica ('shipyard eye'), conjunctivitis follicularis; upper respiratory illness: pharyngitis; pharyngo-conjunctival fever; acute respiratory disease: tracheobronchitis, coryza, pneumonia; gastroenteritis acuta, 'pertussis syndroma', cystitis; central nervous system: meningitis, encephalitis, Reye's syndrome	occurs worldwide as CAI, common in immuncompromised host, occurs as HAI: in ophthalmology and in swimming pools of rehabilitation centres	+
Hepadnaviridae		Orthohepadnavirus	Hepatitis B virus (HBV)	DS DNA	hepatitis acuta, subacuta and chronica, cirrhosis hepatis, hepatocellular carcinoma (HCC), atrophia hepatica flava	occurs worldwide, high occurrence in developing countries, HAI: dentistry, invasive procedures, occupational occurrence	++
Herpesviridae	Alphaher-pesvirinae	Simplexvirus	Human herpesvirus 1 (HHV-1) (formerly herpes simplex virus type 1 or Herpesvirus hominis)	DS DNA	gingivo-stomatitis, encephalitis necrotisans, conjunctivitis, keratitis, Kaposi's varicelliform eruption	occurs worldwide, HAI: important: dentistry (eruption on the hand of dentist), other staff, obstetrics-gynaecology	+
			Human herpesvirus 2 (HHV-2) (formerly herpes simplex virus type 2 or Herpesvirus hominis)	DS DNA	herpes genitalis	sexually transmitted, occurs worldwide	+
		Varicellovirus	Human herpesvirus 3 (HHV-3) (formerly varicella-zoster virus)	DS DNA	varicella (chickenpox), herpes zoster (shingles), encephalomyelitis postinfectiosa, pneumonia	occurs worldwide, HAI: in paediatrics may occur among immuno-compromised patients	+
	Betaherpes-virinae	Cytomegalovirus	Human herpesvirus 5 (HHV-5) (formerly cytomegalovirus)	DS DNA	congenital infection : deafness, mental retardation, chorioretinitis; perinatal infection: neurological disorders; postnatal infection: hepatitis, CMV-enteritis, retinitis, pneumonia, haemolytic anaemia	common in CAI, in HAI: important in recipient of bone marrow and kidney transplantation, HIV patients	++
		Roseolovirus	Human herpesvirus 6 (HHV6) (formerly human B lymphotropic virus)	DS DNA	Roseola (exanthema subitum), encephalitis-encephalopathy, hepatitis	common as CAI in children, occurs as HAI in organ transplantation	+
	Gammaher-pesvirinae	Lymphocryptovirus	Human herpesvirus 4 (formerly Epstein-Barr virus)	DS DNA	mononucleosis infectiosa, Burkitt's lymphoma, carcinoma nasopha-ryngealis	common in CAI, HAI: less important, may occur in paediatrics	+

Family	Subfamily	Genus	Virus	Genome	Disease	Occurrence	
		Rhadinovirus	Human herpesvirus 8 (HHV-8) (formerly Kaposi's sarcoma associated virus)	DS DNA	Kaposi's sarcoma, primary effusion lymphoma (PEL), plasma cell variant of multicentric Castleman's Disease (MCD)	occurs worldwide as CAI	+
Papillomaviridae		Papillomavirus	Human papillomavirus (HPV)	DS DNA	verruca vulgaris (warts), condyloma acuminata, papilloma venereum, neoplasia cervicale, papilloma laryngeale	common in CAI, HAI: less important, but may occur (gynaecology)	+
Parvoviridae	Parvovirinae	Erythrovirus	B19 virus (B19V) (formerly human parvovirus)	SS DNA	erythema infectiosum (formerly fifth disease), haemolysis, influenza-like illness	worldwide occurrence in CAI, HAI: may occur.	+
Poxviridae	Chordo-poxvirinae	Orthopoxvirus	Variola virus	DS DNA	smallpox; variola major (ordinary smallpox, modified smallpox, flat smallpox, haemorrhagic smallpox), variola minor	Eliminated infectious agent. Only laboratory accidents may occur where strains are stored	0
		Molluscipoxvirus	Molluscum contagiosum virus	DS DNA	molluscum contagiosum	sexually transmitted, common in CAI, promiscuous lifestyle	0
Arenaviridae		Arenavirus	Lymphocytic choriomeningitis virus (LCMV)	SS RNA	meningitis, febrile illness	common in CAI	0
			Lassa virus (LASV)	SS RNA	meningo-encephalitis, haemorrhagic fever	Dangerous virus! occurs in West Africa, high lethality, HAI: extremely important in tropics and if imported into other areas	++
Bunyaviridae		Bunyavirus	Bunyaviruses	SS RNA	encephalitis, febrile illness	occurs worldwide as CAI	+
		Hantavirus	Hantaan virus (HTNV)	SS RNA	encephalitis, pneumonia, haemorrhagic fever	occurs worldwide as CAI	+
Caliciviridae		Norwalk-like viruses	Feline calicivirus (FCV)	SS RNA	gastroenteritis acuta	occurs worldwide as CAI	++
			Norwalk virus (NV)	SS RNA	gastroenteritis	occurs worldwide as CAI	++
Flaviviridae		Hepacivirus	Hepatitis C (HCV)	SS RNA	hepatitis acuta et chronica, cirrhosis hepatis, carcinoma hepatocellulare, atrophia hepatica flava	occurs worldwide, higher occurrence in developing countries HAI: very important (patients and occupational aspects)	++
Filoviridae		Marburg-like viruses	Marburg virus (MARV)	SS RNA	Marburg haemorrhagic fever	occurs in central Africa as CAI, dangerous infection	++

Table 1.1. (contd)

Family	Subfamily	Genus	Species	Genome type	Disease	Other characteristics	HAI
Filoviridae		Ebola-like viruses	Reston Ebola virus (REBOV)	SS RNA	Ebola haemorrhagic fever	occurs in central Africa as CAI, dangerous infection	++
			Sudan Ebola virus (SEBOV)	SS RNA	Ebola haemorrhagic fever	occurs in central Africa as CAI, very important as HAI	++
			Zaire Ebola virus (ZEBOV)	SS RNA	Ebola haemorrhagic fever	occurs in central Africa as CAI, very important as HAI	++
Orthomyxo-viridae		Influenzavirus A	Influenza A virus (FLUAV)	SS RNA	influenza, Reye's syndrome, primary influenza pneumonia	occurs worldwide as CAI, pandemic occurrence, HAI; seasonal occurrence from December till April in the Northern hemisphere	++
		Influenzavirus B	Influenza B virus (FLUBV)	SS RNA	same as influenza A	same as influenza A	++
		Influenzavirus C	Influenza C virus (FLUCV)	SS RNA	influenza	localized occurrence in children and young adults	+
Paramyxoviridae	Paramyxo-virinae	Respirovirus	Human parainfluenza virus 1, 3 (HPIV-1, HPIV-3)	SS RNA	coryza, laryngo-tracheobronchitis (croup), bronchiolitis, pneumonia	common as CAI in children	+
			Respiratory syncytial virus (RSV)	SS RNA	coryza, bronchiolitis, pneumonia	very common as CAI worldwide	++
		Morbillivirus	Measles virus (MeV)	SS RNA	morbilli, giant-cell pneumonia, encephalitis or encephalomyelitis postinfectiosa, subacute sclerosing panencephalitis	occurs worldwide and common in countries with low vaccine coverage	+
		Rubulavirus	Mumps virus (MuV)	SS RNA	parotitis epidemica, meningitis, encephalitis, orchitis, pancreatitis, oophoritis (rare), thyroiditis, mastitis, hepatitis, thrombocythopenia	occurs worldwide as CAI	+
			Human parainfluenza virus 2, 4 (HPIV-2, HPIV-4)	SSRNA	coryza, laryngo-tracheobronchitis (croup), bronchiolitis, pneumonia	common as CAI in children	+

Family	Genus	Virus	Nucleic acid	Disease	Epidemiology	Importance
Picornaviridae	Enterovirus	Coxsackie A virus Coxsackie B virus Echovirus Human enterovirus (HEV)	SS RNA	respiratory: herpangina, 'hand-foot-mouth disease', epidemic myalgia (pleurodynia or Bornholm disease); cardiovascular: myocarditis, pericarditis; neurologic: aseptic meningitis, encephalomyelitis, poliomyelitis; conjunctivitis haemorrhagica acuta	occurs worldwide as CAI	+
		Poliovirus (PV)	SS RNA	poliomyelitis acuta, Heine-Medine paralysis, acute flaccid paralysis (AFP)	occurs worldwide as CAI in developing countries where low vaccination coverage, HAI occurs in tropical countries	+
	Hepatovirus	Human hepatitis A (HHAV)	SS RNA	hepatitis epidemica, atrophia hepatica flava (rare)	occurs worldwide as CAI, HAI: due to poor hygiene in tropics	++
	Rhinovirus	Human rhinovirus (HRV)	SS RNA	rhinitis acuta (common cold)	very common as CAI	+
Reoviridae	Rotavirus	Rotavirus (RV)	DS RNA	gastroenteritis	common as CAI worldwide	++
Retroviridae	Deltaretrovirus	Human T-lymphotrop virus (HTLV)	SS RNA	adult T-cell leukemia-lymphoma (ATL)	occurs worldwide as CAI	+
	Lentivirus	Human immundeficiency virus (HIV)	SS RNA	acquired immunodeficiency syndrome (AIDS), Kaposi sarcoma	pandemic as CAI, HAI: occurs if not controlled (developing countries)	++
Rhabdoviridae	Lyssavirus	Rabies virus	SS RNA	rabies (lyssa)	occurs worldwide as CAI	0
Togaviridae	Rubivirus	Rubella virus (RUBV)	SS RNA	rubella, encephalomyelitis postinfectiosa, arthralgia, thrombocytopenic purpura, congenital defects: triad: cataract, nerve deafness, cardiac abnormalities (patent ductus arteriosus, ventricular septal defect, pulmonary artery stenosis, Fallot's tetralogy), and neurologic: microcephaly, meningoencephalitis, and mental retardation	very common as CAI	+

DS = double strained; SS = single-strained; ++ = frequent; + = rare; 0 = not important; CAI = community-acquired infection; HAI = hospital-acquired infection where the particular virus was first discovered (e.g. Crimean haemorrhagic fever virus). The taxonomy of viruses changes, and regular updates of new classifications can be observed (Fauquet and Pringle, 1999; Miller, 1999b).

The Boston classification divides viruses into six main groups according to replication type. It is used for research and anti-viral drug search and production, as the replication can be stopped at different stages of production of virions.

Clinical classification groups together the viruses that cause the same or similar clinical outcome, which is due to the affinity for the same tissue cells. This grouping is important for clinicians in differential diagnosis of viral diseases. However, the same virus can affect different organs leading to an overlap of these groups. The most important groups are:

- respiratory – e.g. flu, parainfluenza, adenovirus
- hepatitis group – e.g. hepatitis A, hepatitis B, hepatitis C, and other hepatitis viruses, cytomegalovirus
- enteric viral disease – e.g. rotavirus, calicivirus
- neurotrop viruses – e.g. rabies, tick-borne encephalitis
- haemorrhagic fever group – e.g. yellow fever, Marburg, Ebola, Lassa
- rash-causing – e.g. measles, German measles, chickenpox, smallpox.

Epidemiological classification is based on the portal of entry of the virus. This is very similar to clinical classification as the main target tissue and portals of entry are usually the same. This system is used for preventive strategies for implementing precautions (see Chapter 3).

Chlamydiae

Chlamydiae are larger micro-organisms than most viruses, their size being about 250–500 nm. They can be seen by a light microscope and contain both DNA and RNA. Like the viruses, they grow only in living cells but the replication cycle is complex, including binary fusion. Chlamydiae are unable to grow on inanimate media, and special tissue cultures are needed for laboratory growth (McCoy or HeLa cells, or the yolk sack of chick embryos).

Chlamydiae are widespread in both humans and animals. Their role in HAI is much less than other micro-organisms, but they may occur in special circumstances and in some geographic regions with poor hygiene, especially in temperate climates. Three species are distinguished, and among them several subtypes can be found, which may cause different or similar infectious diseases (see Table 1.2).

Table 1.2. Characteristics of chlamydia infections in humans

Species	Host	Subtype	Main disease	Other characteristics	HAI
Chlamydia trachomatis	human	A,B,Ba,C	trachoma (follicular conjunctivitis, blindness)	High occurrence in tropical countries, may occur as HAI due to poor hygiene	+
		D–K	neonatal ophthalmia (inclusion blennorrhoea)	occurs in temperate climates among new-borns infected from mother with cervicitis, may occur as HAI due to poor hygiene	+
			inclusion conjunctivitis	children and adults infected indirectly from genitals, or in swimming pools, may occur as HAI due to poor hygiene	+
			urethritis, cystitis, epididymitis, prostatitis, Reiter syndrome (urethritis+arthritis+conjunctivitis), vaginitis, salpingitis, pelvic inflammatory disease (PID)	among males and females mainly sexually transmitted, may occur as HAI due to poor hygiene	+
			pneumonia	mainly among neonates often with conjunctivitis	+
		1,2,3	lymphogranuloma venereum inguinal syndrome in males genito-anorectal syndrome in females	common in tropical countries and unknown in temperate climates, mainly sexually transmitted, may occur as HAI due to poor hygiene	+
Chlamydia pneumoniae (formerly called TWAR, i.e. Taiwan acute respiratory agent)	human	no subtypes	pneumonia sore throat	occurs worldwide as CAI	+
Chlamydia psittaci	animals, human is accidental host	no subtypes	psittacosis	occurs worldwide in community	0

+ = rare; 0 = not important; CAI = community-acquired infection; HAI = hospital-acquired infection

Rickettsiae

Rickettsiae grow and replicate intracellularly by binary fusion, like chlamydiae. Unlike viruses they contain both DNA and RNA and relatively large coccobacilli with a diameter of 300 nm, which can be seen with a light microscope. Accordingly they are classified as bacteria but owing to their special characteristics they are discussed separately. Rickettsial infections occur worldwide, but their occurrence is not uniform across different regions. Two genera belong to the family *Rickettsiae*:

- Rickettsia
- Coxiella.

Rickettsia is transmitted from small animals (e.g. rodents) or from human to human by the bites of arthropods (louse, flea, tick). It is not a common HAI – except *Rickettsia prowazekii* that causes typhus (typhus exanthematicus) as a result of poor infection control in those regions where it occurs in the community. Typhus is an indicator of poverty, poor hygiene and poor infection control because the host of the infection is human. It used to be a major pathogen in wars, where the conditions in camps were appropriate for the infection, and nowadays it can often be found among refugees. Table 1.3 summarizes the main groups of rickettsial infections.

Coxiella burnetii is the only member of the genus Coxiella that has importance for humans but it does not occur as HAI even although it is distributed worldwide. It is common in domestic animals (for example, goats, sheep) and causes Q fever (querry fever) in humans who are infected from contact with animals.

Mycoplasmas

Mycoplasmas are closely related to bacteria but without a rigid cell wall (peptidoglycan) and are able to grow on inanimate bacteriological media. Their size is from 0.1 to 0.2 µm. Two genera are important for humans:

- Mycoplasma
- Ureoplasma.

The third genera – Archeoplasma – are not important in humans.

Mycoplasmas occur worldwide and are one of the most frequent causes of infections in the community, with possible occurrence in hospitals as well. Among them *Mycoplasma pneumoniae* is the most important, causing

Table 1.3. Important rickettsial infections of humans

Genera	Type	Reservoir	Vector	Disease	HAI
Rickettsia	prowazekii	man, flying squirrels (USA)	lice	typhus exanthematicus, Brill–Zinsser disease (recurrent typhus)	+
	typhi	rats	fleas	murine typhus	0
	rickettsii conorii sibirica australis	ticks	ticks	rocky-mountain fever, other 'tick-borne' fevers	0
	akari	mites	mites	'tick-borne' fever	0
	tsutsugamushi	mites	mites	scrub typhus (tsutsugamushi fever)	0
Coxiella	burneti	domestic animals	–	Q-fever	0

+ = rare; 0 = not important; HAI = hospital-acquired infection extensive outbreaks every four or five years in the community. Table 1.4 gives information about mycoplasma infections in humans.

Table 1.4. Important infections in humans caused by mycoplasma

Genera	Types	Disease	Other characteristics	HAI
Mycoplasma	pneumoniae	bronchitis, tracheitis, pneumonia, sinusitis, pharyngitis, coryza, otitis media (myringitis bullosa), Stevens-Johnson syndrome, meningitis or meningo-encephalitis, myelitis, haemolytic anaemia	occurs worldwide as CAI	+
	hominis	urethritis, sepsis neo-natorum, sepsis post-partum	occurs worldwide as CAI	+
	orale	periodontal disease	occurs worldwide, common as CAI	+
	salivarium	periodontal disease	occurs worldwide as CAI	+
	fermentans	respiratory distress syndrome	occurs worldwide as CAI	
Ureoplasma	ureolyticum	urethritis	occurs worldwide as CAI	+

+ = rare; CAI = community-acquired infection; HAI = hospital-acquired infection

Bacteria

Bacteria with cell walls are the most frequent causes of infections, both in the community and in hospitals. They occur worldwide with some variation in different geographic regions. They can grow in a laboratory setting on inanimate media under appropriate conditions (temperature and nutrients). Bacteria multiply by simple cell division (binary) with self-reproduction of DNA and other substances. They can be classified in several ways that are important for their laboratory identification:

- morphological classification
- staining features:
  - Gram stain

- Ziehl-Neelsen technique
- bipolar staining:
  ◦ Albert staining
  ◦ polychromed methylene blue technique
  ◦ Wayson's bipolar staining
- oxygen requirements
- temperature requirements
- spore-producing features.

Morphological classification is important for direct detection of bacteria by light-, electron- or fluorescent microscope. Five main groups of bacteria can be distinguished by morphology:

- cocci – round or oval cells about 0.5 to 1.0 μm in diameter
- bacilli (rods) – stick-like cells with rounded (coccobacilli), tapered, square or swollen ends, 1.0–10.0 μm in length by 0.3–1.0 μm width
- vibrios – slightly curved, motile rods measuring 3.0–4.0 μm in length by 0.5 μm in width
- spirilla – regularly coiled, rigid organisms about 3.0–4.0 μm
- spirochaetes – flexible, coiled, motile organisms measuring 6.0–20.0 μm in length by 0.1–0.5 μm in width.

Staining features of bacteria are connected with the structure of their cell walls and protoplasma, which may adsorb different staining substances, thus helping to distinguish different bacterial groups.

Gram staining is the most frequently used method to stain most of the bacteria of humans. According to the Gram reaction, bacteria can be grouped into Gram-positive and Gram-negative. The differences are thought to be due to differences in the permeability of the cell wall. The cell permeability of Gram-positive bacteria is low and the crystal violet stain treated with iodine remains within the cell (giving a dark purple and sometimes blue colour) even after decolourization with acetone or ethanol. Gram-negative bacteria have high permeability, cannot retain the crystal violet during decolourization and can take neutral red or safranin (giving red) in the last stage of staining. Another explanation is that the acidic protoplasm of Gram-positive bacteria binds the basic stain (helped by iodine), while in Gram-negative bacteria the basic protoplasm cannot bind the basic stain.

Another important difference between Gram-positive and Gram-negative bacteria is that the inner surface of the cell wall of Gram-negative bacteria contains an *endotoxin* that can be released only after the lysis of the cell. If the amount of endotoxin is substantial then it may cause endotoxin shock in humans, with fatal results.

Misclassification of bacteria may happen by Gram stain, i.e. Gram-positive bacteria are stained Gram-negatively and vice versa, for several reasons:

- cell wall damage of Gram-positive bacterium (antibiotic therapy, excess heat fixation)
- over-decolourization (a longer time is taken than is required)
- the iodine solution is not appropriate
- old cell culture
- lack of full decolourization of Gram-negative bacterium.

The Ziehl-Neelsen technique is used to stain those bacteria that do not stain well by the Gram method (*Mycobacteria* including *M. tuberculosis*, *M. ulcerans* and *M. leprae*). The phenolic-carbol fuchsine stain binds to the mycolic acid in the mycobacterial cell (giving a red dye), which cannot be decolourizied by an acid, and is thus referred to as 'acid-fast bacilli' (AFB), while decolourization occurs in the background cells that are stained with methylene blue or malachite in the last phase, providing a blue contrast against which the red AFB can be seen. This is an extremely important method for the prompt diagnosis of tuberculosis if the patient spreads the *Mycobacterium* in the sputum.

Bipolar staining is used for the identification of some rod-form bacteria where the staining dye is accumulated in granules on the opposite side of the bacterium. Polychromed methylene blue is required to stain *Bacillus anthracis* (McFadyean's reaction), which causes a very dangerous disease, anthrax, which can be used as a biological weapon owing to its high lethality. Wayson's bipolar technique is a rapid method to find *Yersinia pestis* (causing plague), while Albert staining is used to stain the volutin or metachromatic granules of *Corynebacterium diphtheriae*, which causes diphtheria.

The *oxygen requirements* for growth provide a further important classification of bacteria:

- aerobes – require free oxygen to grow
- anaerobes – unable to grow in free oxygen

- facultative anaerobes – may grow in the presence or absence of free oxygen
- microaerophiles – grow best in reduced oxygen concentration compared with that of air.

The oxygen dependence of bacteria is important not only for laboratory culture, but also for the development of disease. Anaerobes inhabit the lower part of the gut and may grow only in those tissues where oxygen is absent or minimal due to reduced circulation. Small puncture injuries are the best conditions for anaerobic infections like tetanus or oedema malignum.

The *temperature requirement* is an important feature of bacteria, which defines whether they can survive in the inanimate environment or only in mammals, including humans. In this respect, bacteria can be classified into three main groups:

- psicrophile – growing at lower temperatures (below 10°C)
- mesophile – growing at about 35 – 37°C
- thermophile – growing at high temperature (even at 90°C).

Most human pathogens are mesophile, having adapted to human body temperature.

The *spore-producing feature* of bacteria also determines their ability to survive in extreme climatic situations (heat, dry soil, temperature below zero degrees Celsius, etc.). Spores in soil may survive for years; for example, *Bacillus anthracis* or *Clostridia species*. Their resistance is extremely high against heat and chemicals, thus spores of *Bacillus stearothermophilus* and *Bacillus subtilis* are used to test sterilization procedures (see Chapter 5).

Bacteria account for more than 90% of the causes of HAI, which is associated with their worldwide occurrence. Tables 1.5 and 1.6 summarize the features of the bacteria that have greatest importance in both community and HAI. There are about 15 bacteria that are the most common cause of HAI, but others may occur in different circumstances. Among Gram-positive bacteria, the genera of *Staphylococci*, *Enterococci* and *Clostridia* play an important role in HAI (see Table 1.5).

The Gram-negative bacteria are the major cause of HAI, which can be explained by the relative ease with which they survive in both human and inanimate environments, especially bacteria of the group *Enterobacteriaceae*, *Pseudomonas* and *Acinetobacter* species (see Table 1.6).

Table 1.5. Gram-positive bacteria of importance in hospitals

Morphology	Oxygen requirement	Genera	Type	Disease	Other characteristics	HAI
coccus	aerobe or facultative anaerobe	Staphylococcus	aureus	skin:folliculitis, impetigo, furuncles, scalded skin syndrome, sepsis pneumonia, empyema, osteomyelitis, Staphylococcus toxic shock syndrome (STSS), wound infection, endocarditis, myocarditis, pericarditis, meningitis, abscess in different organs, food-poisoning (produced by enterotoxins)	important in CAI methicillin resistance (MRSA) increasing worldwide and emergence of vancomycin resistance	+++
			epidermidis	wound infections of implants, device-associated bacteraemia, sepsis, meningitis, endocarditis	increasing role in HAIs, not common in community	+++
			saprophyticus	urinary tract infection, wound infection, sepsis	opportunistic pathogen in urinary tract infection of women, but may occur in men	++
		Streptococcus	pyogenes	skin: scarlet fever, toxic shock, impetigo, wound infection, erysipelas, wound scarlet, cellulitis pharyngitis, meningitis, endocarditis, puerperal sepsis, arthritis rheumatoid fever, acute glomerulonephritis	occurs worldwide, important as CAI	++
			agalactiae	meningitis and sepsis in neonates, postpartum infections, sepsis, endocarditis	occurs worldwide as CAI	++
		Enterococcus	faecalis faecium	urinary tract infections, intra-abdominal and pelvic wound infections, bacteraemia, endocarditis, meningitis; tracheobronchitis	occurs worldwide, rare in CAI second most frequent in HAI urinary tract infections; emerge of vancomycin- (VRE) and teicoplanin-resistance	+++
	anaerobe	Peptostreptococcus	prevotii tetradius and other speciei	pelvic infections: postpartum endometritis; abscess of bladder, kidney; orofacial infection: periodontitis, sinusitis, otitis, Pulmonary form: abscess of lungs, pneumonitis, empyema, necrotizing pneumonia	occurs worldwide as CAI	++
rods	aerobic or facultatively anaerobic	Corynebacterium	diptheriae	nasopharingeal and cutaneous diphtheria, myocarditis (caused by toxin strains), non-toxigenic diptheria (endocarditis)	occurs worldwide as CAI especially in unvaccinated	+
			jeikeium	device-associated: endocarditis, meningitis, peritonitis, pneumonia, shunt infections, prosthetic infections	important in HAIs due to devices	+
		Listeria	monocytogenes	meningitis, encephalitis, septicemia, abortion, stillbirth, premature birth	worldwide occurrence as CAI	0

Genus	Species	Diseases	Occurrence	Rating
Nocardia	asteroides amarae and other species	'pseudotuberculosis' (brain), six categories: pulmonary, extrapulmonary, localized, cutaneous-subcutaneous, lymphocutaneous, mycetoma	occurs worldwide especially in immuno-compromised host	+
Mycobacterium	tuberculosis complex (MTC) M. bovis, M. microti, M. africanum	pulmonal: tuberculosis (TB) extra-pulmonal forms: meningitis basillaris, osteomyelitis, renal, skin, pericarditis, synovitis	important as CAI, emergence of multi-resistance, increased occurrence due to HIV and other social factors	++
	avium complex (MAC) 28 serovars	pulmonary disease: solitary nodules, chronic bronchiolitis, tuberculosis-like infiltrates, diffuse infiltrate	occurs worldwide, important as CAI especially in immunocompromised patients and patients with AIDS, multi-resistant feature	++
	leprae	lepra (Hansen's disease)	important in some regions of the world (Asia, Africa) as CAI	0
anaerobe Lactobacillus	several spp	endocarditis, neonatal meningitis, chorioamnionitis, amnionitis, pleuropulmonary infections, bacteremia	occurs worldwide as CAI	++
Propionibacterium	acnes propionicus	acne vulgaris, skin infections associated with operations is increasing, infections of transplants	occurs worldwide as CAI, increasing role in HAI	++
Actinomyces	viscosus naeslundii	cerviofacial: sinusitis, caries, periodontal disease; thoracic: abscess; abdominal: pelvic inflammatory disease associated with intra-uterine devices, pyogenic liver abscess	occurs worldwide as CAI	++
Bacillus	anthracis	cutaneous anthrax, intestinal anthrax, pulmonary anthrax	disease is endemic in many countries among animals, it is a very dangerous microbe (bio-terrorism),	0
	cereus	diarrhoea	food-poisoning, occurs worldwide as CAI, in HAI if catering is not controlled	+
Clostridium	perfringens	oedema malignum, anaerobe cellulitis, pseudomembranosus colitis (antibiotic-associated)	occurs worldwide during injuries as CAI, occurs in surgery, antibiotic associated colitis (produced by toxin A) is important as HAI	++
	botulinum	botulism	occurs worldwide as food-borne disease as CAI, bioterrorism	+
	tetani	tetanus, tetanus neonatorum	occurs worldwide as CAI and in newborns of unvaccinated women as CAI	++

+++ = very frequent (among the top 15); ++ = frequent; + = rare; 0 = not important; CAI = community-acquired infection; HAI = hospital-acquired infection

Table 1.6. Gram-negative bacteria of importance in hospitals

Morphology	Oxygen requirement	Genera	Type	Disease	Other characteristics	HAI
coccus	aerobe	Neisseria	meningitidis	local: pharyngitis, anorectal infection, conjunctivitis, sinusitis disseminated: purulent meningitis, sepsis (meningococcemia), Waterhouse-Friderichsen syndrome, arthritis, endocarditis, primary pneumonia	common as CAI especially in Africa (type C) known as the 'meningitis belt' in sub-Sahara region, but occurs worldwide	+
			gonorrhoeae	urethritis, vulvo-vaginitis, prostatitis, epididymitis, proctitis, pelvic inflammatory disease (PID = endometritis, salpingitis, pelvic peritonitis, tubo-ovarian abscess), conjunctivitis in infants, pharyngitis, disseminated gonococcal infection (DGI): dermatitis-arthritis syndrome, bacteraemia, meningitis	occurs worldwide as sexually transmitted disease as CAI, occurs as HAI in newborns if not controlled	+
rods	aerobe	Pseudomonas	aeruginosa and other species	folliculitis, ecthyma gangrenosum, malignant otitis externa ('swimmer's ear'), meningitis, conjunctivitis, osteomyelitis, endocarditis, chronic lung infection in patients with mucoviscidosis, urinary tract infection, bacteremia, sepsis	one of the most important in CAI and HAI	+++
		Legionella	pneumophila and other species	subclinical infection; pulmonary form: pneumonia; non-pneumonic form: Pontiac fever (fever, malaise, myalgia, cough, flu-like syndrome), enteritis; extrapulmonary form: wound infection	occurs worldwide as CAI associated mainly with air conditioning	++
	facultative anaerobe	Salmonella	typhi	typhoid fever	occurs worldwide as CAI, high occurrence in countries with poor hygiene	+
			enteritidis typhimurium panama and other species	salmonellosis, enteritis, enterocolitis, bacteraemia, abscess, osteomyelitis, empyema	more than 5000 species occur worldwide as CAI (food-borne outbreaks), rarely as HAI (poor hygiene in catering)	+
		Shigella	dysenteriae flexneri boydii sonnei	'bacillary' dysentery or shigellosis	occurs worldwide as CAI, rarely as HAI unless poor personal hygiene	+
		Klebsiella	pneumoniae	bronchopneumonia, lung abscess, urinary tract infection, sepsis, meningtitis	occurs worldwide, emergence of poly-resistance	+++
		Proteus	mirabilis vulgaris and other species	bronchopneumonia, lung abscess, urinary tract infection, sepsis, meningitis; wound infection	occurs worldwide	+++

Genus	Species	Infections/clinical features	Occurrence	
Escherichia	coli	urinary tract infections, cystitis in women; wound infection; peritonitis, sepsis, endotoxin shock, cholecystitis, abscess (brain, etc.); diarrhoeal disease: enterotoxigenic E. coli (ETEC), enteropathogen E. coli (EPEC), enteroinvasive E. coli (EIEC), enterohaemorrhagic E. coli (EHEC)	occurs worldwide, cystitis in women is the commonest as CAI, dyspepsia in newborns is becoming less frequent	+++
Serratia	marcescens	bronchopneumonia, urinary tract infection, wound infection, sepsis, meningitis	recognized as very important hospital pathogen occurring mainly as HAI	+++
Yersinia	pestis	plague	occurs in some geographic regions as CAI, extremely rare as HAI but can be imported to hospitals, bioterrorism	+
	enterocolitica	enterocolitis, terminal ileitis, mesenteric lymphadenitis (pseudoappendicular syndrome), septicemia	common as CAI, occurs worldwide	+
Bordetella	pertussis	pertussis	occurs worldwide in children and elderly people as CAI	+
	parapertussis	parapertussis	occurs worldwide as CAI	+
Haemophilus	influenzae, ducreyi, other species	otitis media, tracheobronchitis, laryngitis, tonsillopharyngitis, pneumonia, conjunctivitis, meningitis, pericarditis, Brazilian purpuric fever	very common as CAI especially among young children	+
Brucella	militensis, abortus, suis, canis	hepatitis, arthritis, arthralgia, osteomyelitis, acute and chronic meningoencephalitis	occurs worldwide as CAI	0
Pasteurella	multocida, canis	wound infection due to animal bites	occurs as CAI worldwide	0
anaerobe Bacteroides	fragilis	traumatic wound infections, intra-abdominal infections: peritonitis; abscess, orofacial infections	occurs worldwide as CAI especially traumatic wound infections, important as HAI	++
Fusobacterium	nucleatum, necrophorum, other species	pharyngotonsillitis, peritonsillar abscess, dissemination: abscess in lungs, liver, large joints, bacteremia (postanginal sepsis syndrome or Lemierre's disease)	occurs worldwide and common as CAI	++
microaerophile Campylobacter	jejuni	enterocolitis, reactive arthritis, bursitis, urinary tract infection, meningitis, endocarditis, peritonitis, erythema nodosum, pancreatitis, abortion, neonatal sepsis, bacteremia	occurs worldwide, common as CAI	+

(contd)

Table 1.6. (contd)

vibrio	aerobe and facultatively anaerobe	Vibrio	cholerae	cholera (secretory diarrhoea)	occurs in India and in other parts of Asia, currently South America due to poor sanitation and water control	+
spirochetes	aerobe	Leptospira	icterohaemorrhagiae	conjunctivitis, pharyngitis, hepatitis, septicemia, meningitis	occurs worldwide as CAI	0
	anaerobe	Borellia	burgdorferi	Lyme disease: erythema migrans, meningoencephalitis, myocarditis, arthritis; erythema cronicum migrans; relapsing fever	occurs worldwide as CAI	0
		Treponema	pallidum	syphilis	occurs worldwide as sexually transmitted CAI	+

+++ = very frequent (among the top 15); ++ = frequent; + = rare; 0 = not important; CAI = community-acquired infection, HAI = hospital-acquired infection

Fungi

Fungi have a more complex eukaryotic cell structure than bacteria because of their differentiation of genetic material into chromosomes. Their cell walls consist of polysaccharides, polypeptides, chitin and the cell membrane, which contains sterols that protect the fungi from antibacterial agents. Most of them can survive independently of humans and animals. Inhalation, ingestion and traumatic implantation are the main mechanisms of fungal infections. Apart from phylogenetic taxonomy, fungi can be further classified by their morphology, replication and clinical features (see Table 1.7).

Morphological classification is the basis for the identification of fungi, and they can be divided into three groups:

- yeasts;
- filamentous fungi or moulds;
- dimorphic.

Yeasts are unicellular round or oval fungi measuring 3.0–15.0 μm. Asexual budding is the method of replication.

Filamentous fungi are multi-cellular, forming branching filaments called hyphae. Moulds reproduce and survive bad conditions by forming conidia and spores.

Dimorphic fungi are able to grow both as yeast (in infected tissues and in the laboratory at 35–37°C) and as moulds (in the soil and in the laboratory at 20 – 30°C).

Clinical classification of fungi is more important in practice, because it reflects the degree of parasitic adaptation and the route by which they enter the host:

- superficial mycoses;
- subcutaneous mycoses;
- systemic mycoses.

Superficial mycoses affect the skin, hair, nails and mucous membrane without invasion of the body. Superficial candidiasis and dermatophytoses belong to this group. Most dermatophytes cannot survive outside the human body, and are thus dependent on host-to-host spread (see Chapter 3).

Subcutaneous mycoses involve the dermis, the subcutaneous tissues and bone as a result of traumatic implantation occurring in rural areas of the tropics and subtropics among people going barefoot.

Table 1.7. The most important fungal infections of humans

Morphology	Genera	Type	Clinical classification				Disease	Other characteristics	HAI
			Cutaneous	Subcutaneous	Systemic				
					True pathogen	Opportunistic			
moulds	Epidermophyton	floccosum	+				tinea corporis, tinea cruris, tinea pedis, tinea manuum	occurs worldwide as CAI	+
	Trichiphyton	rubrum	+				tinea corporis, tinea cruris, tinea pedis	occurs worldwide as CAI	+
		tonsurans	+				tinea capitis	occurs worldwide as CAI	+
	Microsporum	canis	+				tinea capitis, tinea manuum	occurs worldwide as CAI	+
		equinum	+				tinea capitis	occurs worldwide as CAI	+
	Rhizopus	arrhizus	+			+	in immunocompromised patients: forms of mucormycosis: rhinocerebral, craniocerebral; pulmonary, gastrointestinal, disseminated	occurs worldwide as CAI	++
	Rhizomucor	pusillus	+			+	same as Rhizopus arrhizus	occurs worldwide as CAI	++
	Aspergillus	fumigatus flavus niger terreus	+			+	lungs: acute invasive and chronic necrotizing aspergillosis, fungus ball (aspergilloma), tracheo-bronchitis; cerebral aspergillosis; sinusitis; ocular aspergillosis: endophthalmitis, iridocyclitis, viritis; endocarditis; myocarditis; osteomyelitis; cutaneous aspergillosis	occurs worldwide as CAI, common as HAI	+++
yeasts	Cryptococcus	neoformans var. neoformans neoformans	+			+	in patients with T-cell mediated immunological defects and with AIDS:	var. neoformans occurs worldwide	+

Genus	Species	HAI	Clinical features	Occurrence	CAI
	var. gattii, albidus, laurentii	+	meningitis; pulmonary cryptococcosis; cutaneous cryptococcosis: skin abscess, ulcers; osteomyelitis; ocular form: endophthalmitis; prostatitis	var. gattii restricted to tropics and subtropics	++
Candida	albicans, glabrata, tropicalis, parapsilosis	+	oral candidiasis: acute pseudomembranous candidiosis (thrush), acute atrophic candidiosis, chronic atrophic candidiosis (denture stomatitis), chronic hyperplastic candidiosis (Candida leucoplakia) vaginal candidiosis, balanitis; balanoposthitis cutaneous candidiosis (intertrigo), paronychia otomycosis, keratomycosis	occurs worldwide as CAI	+
Scopulariopsis	brevicaulis	+	nail mycosis	occurs worldwide as CAI	+
Malassezia	furfur	+	pityriasis versicolor, Malassezia folliculitis, seborrhoeic dermatitis, sepsis (catheter-related)	occurs worldwide as CAI	+
Blastomyces (dimorphic)	dermatitidis	+	pulmonary blastomycosis, disseminated: cutaneous, osteoarticular, genito-urinary blastomycosis	occurs in North America, Africa	0
Coccidioides (dimorphic)	immitis	+	primary and chronic pulmonary coccidioidomycosis; disseminated: osteomylitis, meningitis	occurs in America, mainly in men and pregnant women, in patients with AIDS	0
Histoplasma (dimorphic)	capsulatum	+	pulmonary form, extra-pulmonary form (central nervous system, adrenal glands, mucocutenous), disseminated	occurs in America, Africa, East Asia, Malaysia	0

+++ = very frequent (among the top 15); ++ = frequent; + = rare; 0 = not important; CAI = community-acquired infection, HAI = hospital-acquired infection.

Systemic mycoses, also referred to as deep mycoses, can be further classified into:

- 'true' pathogens
- opportunistic forms.

True systemic pathogens may invade the host without any predisposing factor, while opportunists spread in an immunocompromised host.

Among fungal infections in hospital, the opportunistic systemic forms are the most frequent, reflecting the concentration of immunocompromised hosts in health care settings (see Table 1.7).

Protozoa

Protozoa are a group of micro-organisms that have various morphological and replication characteristics. Some of them are able to move in the environment by means of different cell structures (e.g. amoebae, flagellates, ciliates). They can be classified by:

- morphology:
  - amoebae
  - flagellates
  - ciliates
  - coccidia
  - microsporidia
- place of habitat in humans:
  - cavities
  - deep tissues or blood.

The phylogeny of *Pneumocystis carinii* has not been determined. It was originally classified with protozoa, but recent observations suggest that it is more closely related to fungi. It causes respiratory illness in patients with severe immunodeficiency, of either congenital or acquired (AIDS) origin. The role of protozoa is important, mainly in community-acquired infections, and their role in hospital acquisition is less than that of other groups (such as bacteria, viruses and fungi), but they do occur. Among them, transfusion-associated malaria should be mentioned in the tropics, where its occurrence is very high (Garfield et al., 1978). Others may also be transmitted in hospital as a result of poor hygiene (see Table 1.8).

Table 1.8. Protozoa having human importance

Habitat	Genera	Type	Disease	Other characteristics	HAI
cavities	Entamoeba	histolytica	intestinal: amoebic colitis (amoebic dysentery), amoebic granuloma (ameboma); extra-intestinal: abscess of liver, lung and brain	occurs worldwide as CAI, very common in tropical and subtropical countries	+
		gingivalis	abscess of lung, gingivostomatitis	occurs worldwide as CAI due to poor oral hygiene	+
	Giardia	lamblia	giardiasis: chronic enteritis, malabsorp-tion, reactive arthritis	occurs worldwide mainly among children	+
	Trichomonas	vaginalis	vaginitis, urethritis, cystitis, prostatitis	occurs worldwide as CAI, common sexually transmitted disease	+
		hominis	non-pathogenic, inhabits the colon	–	0
	Balantidium	coli	colitis (dysentery-like), rarely perito-neal and urogenital invasion	low occurrence world-wide as CAI	+
tissue and blood	Plasmodium	vivax ovale falciparum malariae	malaria	in tropical and sub-tropical countries the most common infection as CAI, very frequent in tropics as HAI	+++
	Toxoplasma	gondii	congenital toxo-plasmosis adults: toxoplasmosis (mononucleosis-like: lymphadenopathy, lymphocythosis); reactivation in AIDS: cerebritis, chorioretinitis, pneumonia, myocarditis	occurs worldwide as CAI, very common	0
	Trypanosoma	gambiense	African trypano-somiasis (sleeping sickness)	occurs in tropical Africa	0

Table 1.8. (contd)

Habitat	Genera	Type	Disease	Other characteristics	HAI
tissue and blood	Trypanosoma	cruzi	American trypano-somiasis (Chagas' disease)	occurs in rural Mexico and Central and South America	0
	Leishmania	tropica	cutaneous and mucosal leishmaniasis	occurs as CAI restricted to India, Pakistan, Middle East, China	0
		donovani	visceral leishmaniasis (Kala-azar)	occurs in tropics and subtropics as CAI	0
	Naegleria	fowleri	primary meningo-encephalitis, granulo-matous amoebic encephalitis	free-living amoebae, occurs worldwide as CAI	0
	Acanthamoeba	castellani	primary meningo-encephalitis, granulo-matous amoebic encephalitis	free-living amoebae, occurs worldwide as CAI	0

+++ = very frequent; + = rare; 0 = not important, CAI = community-acquired infection; HAI = hospital-acquired infection

Helminths (worms)

Helminths have a role in human infections – mainly in tropical and sub-tropical countries where their occurrence in the community is high because of climatic and poor hygiene factors. Their role in developed countries with temperate climates is getting less and less; however, there is always a possibility of their being introduced by travellers. Their occurrence in hospitals is rare, but some can be transmitted if infection control is poor, and laboratory workers can also be infected if they do not observe the laboratory safety regulations.

Helminths are complex organisms, measuring from 1.0 mm to 10.0 m. They undergo a complex life cycle to achieve the mature stage: eggs – intermediate stages (larvae) – mature helminth – eggs. They can replicate asexually or sexually. Helminths infect humans via ingestion or penetratation of the skin (larvae). The appropriate form – called the infective form – is needed for successful infection. Helminths live in the intestine, liver duct or in the deep tissues of humans, causing different diseases (mechanical obstruction in the intestine and ducts, malnourishment, toxic effect and allergy). Two systems are used to classify helminths:

- biological
- epidemiological.

Biological classification relies on the morphology of the mature worm, which can be:

- flat worms:
  - unsegmented (flukes)
  - segmented (tapeworms)
- cylindrical worms.

Flukes are unsegmented, flat, leaf-like worms without a body cavity. In humans only the adult form is found. About 10 flukes have important consequences for humans: *Clonorchis sinensis, Opisthorchis viverrini, Fasciola hepatica, Fasciolopsis buski, Metagonimus yokogawai, Paragonimus westermani, Schistosoma haematobium, Schistosoma mansoni, Schistosoma intercalatum, Schistosoma japonicum.*

Tapeworms are segmented and tape-like without a body cavity. They obtain nutrients through their body surface. Tapeworms, except the *Echinococcus*, live in the human intestine. The following tapeworms are important for humans: *Taenia solium, Taenia saginata, Echinococcus granulosus, Echinococcus multilocularis, Hymenolepis nana, Diphillobohrium latum, Spirometria* species.

Cylindrical worms (nematodes) have a body cavity and a cuticle (skin). For most of them humans are the only host. Their life cycle is also complex, passing through several stages. The following nematodes are important for humans: *Ascaris lumbricoides, Toxocara canis, Enterobius vermicularis, Strongiloides stercoralis, Strongiloides füelleborni, Trichuris trichiura, Ancylostoma duodenale, Necator americanus, Wuchereria bancrofti, Loa loa, Onchocerca volvulus, Dracunculus medinensis, Trichinella spiralis, Brugia* species, animal hookworms.

Epidemiological classification is important because it classifies worms according to the means of infection of humans:

- biohelminths
- geohelminths
- contact helminths.

Biohelminths infect humans by the ingestion of animal food products containing the infective form for humans. For example, pork containing

Taenia solium or beef infected with *Taenia saginata*. Others are: *Trichinella spiralis, Diphillobothrium latum.*

Geohelminths infect humans by means of *soil* containing the infected form (eggs or larvae). Among them are: *Ascaris lumbricoides, Trichuris trichura, Toxocara canis, Ancylostoma duodenale.*

Contact helminths are transmitted by direct contact from person to person and they may have importance in HAI, as a result of poor hygiene and negligence of hand washing, because they are spread by faeces and infection occurs by ingestion. The following are important: *Taenia solium* (can also be biohelminth), *Enterobius vermicularis, Strongiloides stercoralis, Hymenolepis nana.*

Medical staff should be familiar with the epidemiological classification of worms and should avoid direct contact with faeces (by wearing gloves), and laboratory workers should be aware of the danger if they perform any faecal analysis. If direct contact happens then careful hand washing and disinfection is needed to prevent infection. It should be emphasized that faeces are also a dangerous source of other infections.

Arthropods (insects)

Arthropods of importance to human health are also called 'ectoparasites' and live on the outer surface (skin, hair) of humans. Their life cycle needs animal or human blood, which they obtain from the blood vessels of the skin. In humans they are important in two respects:

- 'true' parasites:
  - louse – pediculosis
  - itch – scabies
- vectors – transmitting other infectious agents:
  - mosquitoes:
    - *Plasmodia* (malaria)
    - viruses – e.g. yellow fever
  - ticks:
    - viruses – e.g. tick-borne encephalitis
    - *Rickettsia*
  - lice:
    - *Rickettsia*
  - flies:
    - *Shigella*
    - *Onchocerca*
    - *Loa.*

'True parasites' cause several diseases by direct tissue invasion, envenomation, vesication and hypersensitivity. Their presence in the tissues of the skin may lead to secondary bacterial infections. Many ectoparasites, being vectors, are able to transmit infectious agents mechanically or biologically (see Chapter 3).

Arthropods occur worldwide. Lice living on humans are indicators of poor human hygiene because humans are their only host. Ticks and mosquitoes may survive in the environment sharing humans and animals in blood taking, and have geographical and climatic occurrence.

The role of arthropods in hospitals should not be ignored because patients with poor hygiene may be admitted and be a source of infection. Patients infected with ectoparasites put the staff and other patients at risk of infection.

Normal microbial flora of humans

Micro-organisms living on the surfaces and in the cavities of the human body are referred to as 'normal flora'. Normal microbial human flora consist of bacteria and fungi (see Table 1.9).

Microbial flora are able to live on and in humans as a result of the mutual adaptation of these micro-organisms and humans to each other. Some of them synthesize vitamin K, or take part in the conversion of bile pigments and acids, while others may cause disease (see Tables 1.5, 1.6 and 1.7).

The normal flora of admitted patients change during hospitalization and are replaced by the flora circulating in the hospital, which can be more resistant to anti-microbial agents (Johanson et al., 1969).

Microbiological diagnosis of infections

Micro-organisms cannot be seen by the naked eye (except helminths and ectoparasites), and so we need special microbiological methods to identify the presence of a micro-organism in the inanimate environment and in a human host. Microbiological identification means defining the taxonomic position of a particular micro-organism obtained from the host up to species or subspecies level. Microbiological methods can be classified into two main groups:

- identification methods:
  - culture methods
  - non-culture methods
- serological methods.

Culture methods are used to provide the appropriate circumstances for a micro-organism to replicate and grow in a laboratory setting. Culturing enables small or inadequate quantities of micro-organism in the specimens to be increased to useful levels. Tissue cells (for viruses, rickettsia, chlamydia) or inanimate media (for mycoplasma, bacteria, fungi) are used as growth media for this purpose. Another aim is to conserve the cultured strain for further practical (anti-microbial resistance, typing, toxin production) and scientific use (e.g. gene mapping, etc.). Two conditions are required to achieve successful culture:

- Micro-organisms in the collected specimen must be viable.
- The ability to grow and replicate in a laboratory setting must be present.

Microbiological identification by the culture method needs an appropriate timescale because the speed of replication of different micro-organisms is not the same. Fast-growing micro-organisms may achieve an adequate amount within 48 hours (most vegetative bacteria), while slow-growing ones may need several days (e.g. anaerobic bacteria, fungi, viruses) or even several weeks (e.g. *Mycobacteria*). This limits the availability of the microbiological results in urgent cases, and clinicians should take into account the earliest date when the result will be obtainable.

The culture method is also called 'isolation', which should not be confused with the 'isolation of infection' used to prevent the spread of a micro-organism in the environment (see Chapter 5). The population of a micro-organism obtained from a specimen via the culture method is called the 'primary strain' to distinguish it from later populations obtained by repeated culture. The number of microbial units produced by *one* viable unit (cell, virion) at the beginning of the culture may attain 10^8 viable particles in such a population. Micro-organisms may change during repeated culture, which is the basis of the attenuation of the pathogen strains for live vaccine production (see Chapter 5). Isolated strains can survive being frozen down to minus 70° C, making it possible to do later research while conserving the biological characteristics of the primary isolation strain.

Non-culture methods rely on the direct detection of a micro-organism in the specimen. In most cases the result may be obtained on the same day that the specimen is collected, or within two days at most, and it is an excellent method in urgent cases. Direct detection is done by visual inspection of a micro-organism, or its specific structures if possible, to identify its species by its morphological features (shape, size, cell accessories, etc.). Apart from the

Table 1.9. The normal microbial flora of humans

Micro-organism	Skin	Mucosa						Gastrointestinal tract	
		Mouth and oropharynx	Outer ear	Conjunctivae	Nose	Urethra	Vagina	Small intestine	Large intestine
Staphylococci coagulase-negative	+	+	+	+	+	+			+
Staphylococcus aureus	+	+		+	+				+
Streptococci viridans		+			+				
Streptococcus pneumoniae		+			+				
Streptococci β-hemolytic (non A group)		+							
Streptococci various species	+			+		+	+		+
Enterococci								+	+
Peptostreptococcus spp.						+	+		+
Diphtheroids	+	+	+			+	+		
Propionibacterium acnes	+								
Mycobacterium spp.	+					+		+	+
Gardnerella vaginalis							+		
Lactobacillus spp.							+	+	+
Bacillus spp	+								
Clostridium spp.							+	+	+
Actinomyces spp.		+							+
Neisseria spp.		+			+				
Branchamella catarrhalis		+							
Pseudomonas spp.			+						+
Acinetobacter spp.									+
Escherichia coli			+					+	+
Klebsiella spp.			+					+	+
Proteus spp.			+					+	+
Haemophilus spp.		+		+	+				
Veillonella spp.		+							
Eikenella corrodens		+							
Treponema spp.		+							
Bacterioides spp.		+				+	+	+	+
Fusobacterium spp.		+				+			+
Candida spp.	+	+					+		
Malassezia furfur	+								

quick result, the main advantage of the direct method is that even *non-viable* microbes can be detected in the specimen. Another advantage of the direct method is the possibility for the clinician to make a judgement about the possible cause of an infection much earlier than by the culture method, which is extremely important for the first choice of anti-microbial agents. However, its main disadvantage is that the strain cannot be isolated, which limits its further microbiological analysis, and its storage is not feasible. Six main types of direct detection are used:

- inspection by eye
- native wet preparation
- stained smear
- antigen test
- fluorescent method
- molecular biological methods.

Inspection by eye can be done only with some helminths that can be distinguished by their biological morphology. For example, it is easy to recognize *Ascaris lumbricoides* in faeces.

Native wet preparation is used if the morphological characteristics of a micro-organism can be clearly seen in a light microscope (for example, *Giardia lamblia*). If the specimen is too viscous it is diluted to make it possible for the investigator to detect the microbes under the microscope.

A *stained smear* is prepared if a micro-organism can be detected or identified better by its specific staining features than by native wet preparation. It is the most widely used method in bacteriology, mycology and parasitology. Stained smear is a complementary method to the culture methods for bacteria and fungi, and is used for the microbiological differentiation of these microbes, but there are some infections where stained smear is the only way to confirm the type of the microbe (e.g. *Plasmodia* in malaria). The staining method is usually able to characterize the affiliation of the given micro-organism at group or family level, and in some cases at species level (e.g. *Plasmodia*). For example, Gram stain differentiates bacteria by the permeability of the cell wall, grouping them into Gram-positive and Gram-negative but without specification of the species. However, it provides extremely valuable information in bacterial infections, especially if the culture fails to detect the bacterium. In this case the clinician's diagnosis can rely only the result of the stain smear (see Tables 1.5 and 1.6).

An *antigen test* is the detection of the antigens of micro-organisms by immunological reaction, where the micro-organism-specific antibody reacts to its specific antigens. Different types of antigen test have been developed; among them the most common is agglutination, which is a production of visible coagulant on a plate (plate agglutination) or in a tube (tube agglutination). The antigen test is rapid if it done directly with the specimen, for example, the rapid detection of *Haemophilus influenzae*, *Nesseria meningitidis* or *Streptococcus pneumoniae* in liquor. Another example is the detection of *Rotavirus* in faeces by latex agglutination. This method is also used for the identification of the cultured strain, which relies on the species-specific antigens. For example, identification of *Salmonella* by O and H antigens by agglutination.

The *fluorescent method* is used to detect and identify micro-organisms using a fluorescent microscope. The specimen is stained with fluorochrome – a dye that is able to transform the invisible ultraviolet light into visible light (just-visible deep blue, yellow or orange) – making the cells glow (fluoresce) against a dark background. This method is widely used for the diagnosis of malaria, trypanosomes, acid-fast bacilli, gonococci, meningococci, etc. Immunofluorescence is a subtype of this method, when fluorochrome attaches to the antigen–antibody complex of cells treated with a specific antibody, which is common in virus diagnostics.

Molecular biological methods are the newest very rapid diagnostic methods in microbiology. Their essence is the detection of the *gene sequence* in the specimen that is specific to a species. The discovery of the polymerase chain reaction (PCR) was a revolution in molecular biology because even one piece of target gene sequence can be replicated by a thermonuclease enzyme and millions of gene 'offspring' can be produced within a day. The population of gene offspring can be made visible by other test (gels, chromatography, etc.) confirming the presence of the microbe's genes. The test can detect even non-viable micro-organisms. The method can also be used to detect the genes responsible for resistance against anti-microbial agents. For example, detection of the mecA gene in methicillin-resistant *Staphylococcus aureus* (MRSA) (Archer and Pennell, 1990).

Serology is the detection of antibodies produced by the host – an indirect method of microbiological diagnosis, which is also an immunological method. Here specific known antigens are used to detect antibodies called immunglobulins (Ig) of class IgM or IgG in the sera of the host. That is why the method is called 'serology'. The advantage of this method is that – if the quantity of antibodies is enough, and lasts for long enough – earlier and more recent infections can be distinguished. Presence of IgM confirms that the infection was acquired not later than 6–8 weeks before the blood was taken. The presence of IgG may show earlier and more recent infections, according to the dynamic of its titre. Raising the titre (at least fourfold) of IgG between two samples of sera taken at an interval indicates recent infection, while lack of change in the titre indicates earlier infection. Serology is a common diagnostic approach to infectious diseases, especially in viral infections. However, many micro-organisms do not initiate the production of antibodies detectable by these methods (e.g. *Staphylococcus aureus*), so limiting the use of this method to identify certain groups of micro-organisms. It is a challenge to microbiology to refine serology in order to find such species-specific substances in the host to promote a wider range of microbiological identification.

Diagnosis of clinical infection and screening

As we have seen, microbiology tries to identify microbes in both the animate and inanimate environments. Two main purposes for a microbiological investigation can be distinguished:

- clinical diagnosis
- screening.

The aim of clinical microbiology is to confirm the aetiology of recent clinical infections in humans, or past infections.

Screening in medicine is done in order to detect by laboratory or image diagnostic methods a health-related event in an individual that is not detectable by other methods owing to the lack of clinical signs. Screening has two main purposes:

- disease-oriented
- microbiological.

Disease-oriented screening is done to detect a disease in its early stages in order to avoid serious consequences or early death by applying prompt treatment (e.g. phenylketonuria in newborns, breast cancer or cervix cancer in women, etc.).

Microbiological screening is carried out in order to identify the recent or past presence of a micro-organism in a host showing no clinical signs. Microbiological screening is not restricted to the animate environment (animals or humans) but is also important for finding potential sources of micro-organisms in the inanimate environment. Any of the microbiological methods (identification or serology) can be used after taking appropriate specimens from the host or from the inanimate environment. The aims of screening are:

- to find potential 'silent' sources of a micro-organism
- to discover the proportion of a population that has been infected with a microbe
- for quality control in water supply, the food industry, pharmaceutical industry, etc.

Microbiological screening can be divided into:

- general
- targeted.

General microbiological screening is done to detect a group of, or all the possible, micro-organisms with which a human has been infected. For example, it is advisable to screen travellers for parasite or helminth infections after returning home from tropical countries. Another example is the bacteriological screening of patients transferred from one hospital to another. Regular general screening is done to check the bacteriological safety of drinking water at water supply companies. Such a diagnostic method is chosen so that many species of microbes may be detected in a specimen at the same time.

Targeted microbiological screening aims to detect a particular microbe, for example HIV screening of blood donors. The laboratory method chosen is specific to a particular micro-organism. Another example is the MRSA screening of patients and staff in hospitals to identify all possible sources.

Principles of specimen collection and transport for microbiology

The available microbiological methods – apart from scanning microscopy – are unable to detect micro-organisms directly in the environment. This forces us to take specimens by means of a sampling procedure. Different micro-organisms have different survival rates in the inanimate environment, which may result in premature death of the microbe in the specimen, hence making it impossible to detect it. Temperature and humidity are the most important factors for survival. Mesophil micro-organisms (e.g. *Neisseria meningitidis*) rarely survive at room temperature (20–25°C) or below, which means that the microbiological identification must commence immediately after the specimen is taken. The ideal would be to move the microbiological laboratory to the place where the particular micro-organism of interest occurs or alternatively to take the sample from the host in the laboratory. However, in practice this is not always feasible, and it is necessary to transport the collected specimens to the laboratory. In some cases transport is not possible; for example, if we want to detect vegetative forms of *Entamoeba histolytica* (a mesophil protozoan) in faeces from a host in a temperate climate it is necessary to produce the faeces close to the laboratory because the detection process must begin within minutes.

The appropriate collection and transport of specimens is the responsibility of clinical staff and those who are charged with the task. The collection and transport of specimens to the microbiological laboratory entails special requirements if the microbiological investigation to be successful. This is a part of the overall quality control of a microbiological investigation and it involves several consecutive steps (see Figure 1.2).

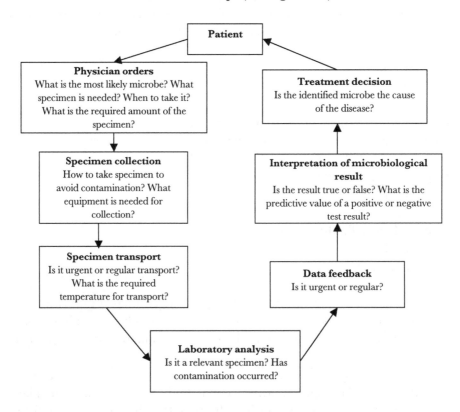

Figure 1.2. The process and quality assurance of a microbiological investigation.

When collecting specimens the following factors should be taken into account:

- the type of specimen
- the quantity required
- the method of collection
- the frequency and time of collection
- transport.

The *type of specimen* to be collected depends on the occurrence of the particular micro-organism and whether an identification or serological method is to be used for the microbiological diagnosis. The most important point is that the clinician should formulate a preliminary hypothesis about the expected micro-organism according to the observed pathological process. If a specimen is collected for screening and the identification method is used, then such a specimen should contain the maximum possible quantity of the micro-organism. For serology blood should be collected, while for the identification method several types of specimen should be collected at the same time:

- body fluids
- tissue.

Body fluids are those fluids that circulate in the body or are excreted by different organs. They can be classified into two main groups:

- physiological fluids:
  - sterile
  - non-sterile
- pathological fluids:
  - sterile
  - non-sterile.

Sterile physiological fluids do not normally contain micro-organisms, and culture of any micro-organism from such a source indicates an infection if contamination can be excluded (blood, cerebrospinal, synovial, pericardial).

Non-sterile physiological fluids, excreted from the body, contain normal flora (sputum, tears, saliva, faeces, urine, vaginal fluid). Such specimens are likely to contain micro-organisms in healthy people. Thus a positive culture confirms an infection, but the interpretation of the result – whether to regard the isolated micro-organism as a pathogen or not – depends on the clinical picture and the type of the isolated microbe. The cultured micro-organism may or may not belong to the normal flora, which helps in the decision-making, but we have to bear in mind that the bacteria of normal flora also *may* cause a clinical infection (see Tables 1.5, 1.6 and 1.9). It is a great mistake for the microbiological laboratory to report that 'normal microflora have been cultured' instead of reporting the presence of specific microbes. All isolated microbes – except those from faeces – belonging to the normal flora should be reported individually because it cannot be decided in the laboratory whether a microbe of normal flora is the cause of an infection or not.

Sterile pathological fluids are those that are produced during non-infectious pathological processes, and they are produced by pure mechanical filtration, known as transudation (ascites, hydrocele). They should be free of any micro-organisms. Presence of a microbe in the ascites may reflect spontaneous bacterial peritonitis. Contamination should also be excluded.

Non-sterile pathological fluids are those that are produced by inflammation due to infection (pus, serous, fibrinous). Here we should expect the presence of a micro-organism causing the pathological process.

The *quantity of specimen* required is determined by the laboratory method for the proper analysis of the specimen. However, in practice it is not always possible to collect the minimal amount owing to individual circumstances and a smaller quantity of the specimen is obtainable than is required. The type and amount of specimen required determines the method of collection. The general principle is: the more of the specimen that is collected the easier it is to do microbiological tests, especially if more than one test is required from the same specimen or if the test has to be repeated for some reason. Each test has its own minimal specimen size to carry out the test properly. Serology needs a minimum of 1–2 ml sera depending on the type of test, which normally presents no problems to collect.

The *method of collection of specimen* depends on one or more of the following factors:

- the preliminary decision about the expected type of micro-organism
- the type of specimen required
- the minimum quantity of specimen needed.

The general principle of any collection is that microbial contamination should be avoided. Any such contamination may affect the microbiological diagnosis, leading to false positive results. This is especially important if the diagnosis is to be made using the culture technique. Appropriate labelling (the name of the person from whom the specimen was collected, identification number, date of collection, type of specimen, the name of the collector, preliminary clinical diagnosis, suspected micro-organism) is important information for the microbiologist and for interpretation of the result.

It is advisable for the clinician to formulate a preliminary idea of all the possible micro-organisms for which the specimen needs to be tested because the type of specimen, the amount and the method of collection will depend on this. Consultation with an infectologist or clinical microbiologist is important at this stage.

Tissue specimens are usually collected by a biopsy technique (for skin and deep tissues) or through an operation by an incision method (for deep tissues). If different tests are scheduled (e.g. for histology and microbiology) then at least two pieces of specimen tissue are needed.

In the case of body fluids the method of collection depends on the amount of fluid required:

- by container:
  - empty
  - with a transport medium
- by swab:
  - dry
  - with a transport medium.

An *empty container* is used if the specimen to be collected is more than 2 ml, which can apply to cerebrospinal fluid, large abscesses, ascites, large exudates, and blood for both culture and serology.

The *swab technique* is used if the amount to be collected is less than 2 ml. The essence of a swab is that cotton, Dacron (polyester) or calcium alginate are rolled around the end of a wooden, metallic or plastic stick, which sucks up the fluid together with any micro-organism. The user should consult the local microbiological laboratory about which type of swab to use because the survival of micro-organisms varies among the different types of swabs (Miller, 1999a, p. 9).

Transport media serve to promote the survival of micro-organisms, and are of two types according to their consistency:

- liquid-based
- gel format.

A liquid-based medium is used if the body fluid is collectable by container or swab. Its advantage is that some drops of body fluid may be adequate if the culture technique is used for bacteria. Swabs can be immersed in the liquid transport medium. The gel format is also used for both the container and swab techniques.

Transport media can also be classified according to the function of the medium:

- preserving
- enriching
- selective.

Preserving transport media try to keep the micro-organism alive in the same form and quantity as at the time of collection. No additional growth occurs and they may inhibit the growth of contaminant microbes.

Enriching transport media promote the replication of those micro-organisms that can grow on inanimate media.

Selective transport media promote the preservation or growth of only a particular micro-organism, while inhibiting the growth of contaminants.

Different transport media have to be used for different micro-organisms, thus the preliminary assumption about the possible micro-organism is important in choosing the transport medium. Some bacteria, such as anaerobes, can be cultured only if the specimen is collected in a transport medium or a container that excludes air because the normal oxygen concentration of air may inhibit the growth of these bacteria. As a result of advanced microbiological technology more and more transport media are available and it is advisable to collect all specimens in appropriate transport media where microbiological identification relies on the culture technique.

The *time of collection* of specimens should be in accordance with the flow of the infectious process in individuals (see Chapter 2). The time of collection is optimal if the specimen allows detection of the infection at the highest sensitivity of the test. The sensitivity of the test depends strongly on the number of microbial or antibody particles in the specimen. The number of microbial particles is usually highest during the shedding or invasion of a microbe in the host. The maximum level of antibody production may vary for different infections, but usually achieves the detectable level on the fifth day after the starts of clinical infection, but for some infections – e.g. HIV or hepatitis C – about one month or even later.

The *frequency of collection* may increase the diagnostic sensitivity, especially if the microbiological diagnosis depends on identification methods, because the shedding and invasion of micro-organisms may vary from day to day. This is important if the microbiological test is negative but where there is still a strong assumption that the patient has an infection.

The *transport of specimens* from the place of collection to the laboratory should be done as quickly as possible. The role of quick transport cannot be overestimated because the microbes must survive in the specimen until the initiation of the microbiological test. Drying should be avoided because microbes do not tolerate it, which results in a false negative result. The general rule is that – except for serology – all specimens should arrive in the laboratory within one hour or less after collection; for protozoa this time is even less – in the case of fresh stools within 30 minutes. Microbiological testing should begin immediately upon the specimen arriving at the laboratory, especially in culture methods. It should be emphasized that the use of transport media is not a reason for delay. Very few rapid techniques are used in routine microbiology, so any delay in transport will prolong the microbiological identification, leading to the late availability of the results. Treatment of many infectious diseases is time-dependent, so late microbiological results may cause inappropriate anti-microbial treatment and preventive measures, which may entail treatment at additional cost, and may even result in loss of life.

The interpretation of microbiological results

The interpretation of microbiological results is the last step in the process of microbiological diagnosis, and is usually the task of the clinicians or those who requested the microbiological test (see Figure 1.2). There are strict rules of interpretation, which are important for both clinical and infection control practice. The most important is whether the test result is true, regardless of whether it is positive or negative. The terms 'positive' and 'negative' result can be applied in two ways:

- dichotomous
- nominal categorical.

A *dichotomous result* occurs when the test aims to detect a particular microbe and the result can have only *two* alternatives – yes or no; for example, the presence of HIV antibodies in the sera, or the presence of *Mycobacteria* in the sputum by acid-fast stain.

A *nominal categorical result* occurs when the test is not specific for a particular microbe, and it may have detected other micro-organisms at the same time, thus many alternative positive results can be expected. For example, a culture medium may detect both *Staphylococcus aureus* and *Streptococcus pyogenes*. Furthermore, in the case of mixed infection more than one micro-organism should be found in the specimen. A false positive result occurs if a microbial species occurring in the specimen is identified as *another* that was not present in the original specimen.

Misclassification occurs if the 'observation test' describes the 'reality' falsely (see Table 1.10). This is one of the most important factors in the interpretation of any diagnostic test.

The result of a microbiological diagnosis in terms of true or false results may depend crucially on the collection, the transport or the microbiological test itself. Microbiological testing has objective (technical circumstances) and subjective (the knowledge and experience of the microbiologist) elements that influence the final result. Misclassification of cases may occur in the following situations:

- depending on the laboratory test:
  - sensitivity of the test
  - specificity of the test
- independent of the sensitivity and specificity of the laboratory test:
  - if the specimens of two patients are exchanged during the:
    - collection
    - laboratory analysis
  - inappropriate collection of the specimen:
    - type
    - amount
    - time
  - contamination during:
    - specimen collection
    - transport
    - laboratory investigation.

The most common cause of misclassification of cases is the inadequacy of laboratory testing.

A *sensitivity-dependent false negative result* occurs if the sensitivity of the laboratory test is less than 100%. Sensitivity is defined as the proportion of *true* cases found by the test from among those cases that are present in reality. Sensitivity depends on the ability of the test to detect the substance (microbe or antibody) in the specimen or the subjective ability of the microbiologist

Table 1.10. Misclassification of the reality by an observational test

Observational test	Reality		Total
	presence of an event	absence of an event	
finds the presence of an event	number of presenting cases where the test can detect the presence of an event (true positive result)	number of false cases where the test detects a non-existent event (false positive result)	total number of cases (true and false positive) where the test finds the presence of an event
finds the absence of an event	number of cases where the test cannot detect an event that is present in reality (false negative result)	number of cases where the test is able to confirm the absence of an event (true negative result)	total number of cases (both true and false negative) where the test cannot detect the presence of an event
Total	total number of cases (true positive and false negative) where the event is present in reality	total number of cases (false positive and true negative) where the event does not exist in reality	total number of cases where the event is present or absent

in microbiological analysis or reading the test. For example, culture methods are not able to detect all the micro-organisms in a specimen because non-viable micro-organisms will not grow even though they are present in the specimen.

A *specificity-dependent false positive result* occurs if the specificity of the laboratory test is less than 100%. Specificity is defined as the proportion of true negative cases found by the test among those cases where the event is absent in reality. Contamination is the most important factor to be taken into account in the interpretation of culture results. In case of serology the 'hypersensitive' method is used initially to screen blood for HIV, which may give false positive results. However, it is vital not to miss even one case of HIV-positive blood by avoiding false negative results. This results in low specificity. However, in the second round of testing all HIV-positive blood is tested with several highly specific tests in order to confirm the true positive results, and to withdraw the false positive results apparent in the first round.

Clinicians should consult the microbiologist about the sensitivity and specificity of microbiological methods used. However, in practice, *predictive values* are more useful in evaluating both positive and negative results.

The *predictive value of positive test* (PVPT) is the second important measure of the interpretation of a positive result, which is the proportion of true positive cases found by the test among all positive cases (true plus false) found by the test. For example, if PVPT is 70% then three positive results are false out of ten, i.e. only seven results are real (true) positive.

The *predictive value of negative test* (PVNT) is used to interpret a negative result, which is defined as the proportion of true negative cases found by the test among all negative cases (true plus false) found by the test. For example, if PVNT is 60%, then four negative results are false among ten negative results given by the laboratory.

It would be desirable to develop diagnostic tests with a sensitivity and specificity of 100%. However, often an increase in the sensitivity leads to a decrease in the specificity, and vice versa. Tests used in practical clinical laboratories are quite different from those used in research or in reference laboratories, for several reasons (cost, ease of performing the test, time required, etc.). Quality control of microbiological laboratories should consist of the benchmarking of reliability and validity of their tests against standard reference tests (called 'the gold standard'), which usually have higher sensitivity and specificity. However, if the reference tests have a sensitivity and specificity lower that 100% some uncertainty will always remain in the diagnostic procedure.

Misclassification may be caused by factors *other* than laboratory sensitivity and specificity. Therefore, staff carry the same responsibility to avoid false results. Sensitivity-independent false negative results can occur by inaccurate labelling causing specimens to be attributed to the wrong patient, by inappropriate methods of collection, or by delays in transport. Specificity-independent false positive results can also caused by the mislabelling of specimens, or by contamination of the specimen at the collection, transport or laboratory investigation stage.

Typing and the principles of molecular epidemiology

Typing is defined as the determination of the clonal difference between identified microbes that is due to the mutations (changes in the nucleic acid sequence) in their genetic material during replication, which may lead to the difference in phenotype features among strains. Clone: 'A population of cells or organisms derived from a single cell or organism by asexual or vegetative propagation'. The word is of Greek origin: *klōn* = a young shoot (Churchill's, 1989, p. 380). The genetic diversity of microbes depends on the stability of the genome within a species. Isolates are epidemiologically related if they come from the clonal expansion of a single precursor.

Molecular clock is the expression used to describe the rate of substantial change in the genome that leads to the divergence in the clonal expansion. The speed of the molecular clock defines the diversity of isolates within a species at a given point in time. It can be used to determine the speed of evolution.

Molecular epidemiology is the common term introduced to investigate the difference in epidemiological and clinical behaviour of micro-organisms using immunology, biochemistry and genetic methods (Maslow et al., 1993). Molecular epidemiology has been used for four main purposes of practical importance:

- phylogenetic characterization of micro-organisms (taxonomy and evolution)
- global spread of clones
- studying transmission within a limited time and space:
  - outbreak investigation
  - association between individual cases
  - finding the source of the infection
- pathogenicity:
  - virulence factors
  - resistance factors.

Typing methods differ and their relative usefulness is assessed by a comparison of the 'type-ability' (performance of the test with each isolate), discriminatory power (the ability to distinguish one clone from another), reproducibility (obtaining the same result if it is repeated on the same isolate), ease of performance and interpretation, availability, and cost (Maslow et al., 1993; Maslow and Mulligan, 1996).

Two sorts of typing methods have been developed:

- phenotying
- genotyping.

Phenotype methods are classical typing and they rely on the investigation of the external features of the micro-organism. However, different clones may show the same phenotype and, alternatively, strains belonging to the same clone may not express the same phenotype characteristic. The following phenotype methods are used:

- biotyping – biochemical reactions
- biocin-typing – biocin production
- antibiotic resistance pattern
- bacteriophage typing – lysis of bacterium cell caused by a virus known as a bacteriophage
- serotyping – serological reactions
- polyacrylamide gel electrophoresis (PAGE) – separation of cellular and membrane proteins
- multilocus enzyme electophoresis (MLEE) – mobility of metabolic enzymes.

Phenotyping is used for limited purposes – outbreak investigation or pathogenicity studies – owing to its relatively low discriminatory power. However, the results of different isolates from different sources cannot be comparable among different laboratories at different times unless the methods are standardized.

Genotyping methods are based on studying the similarities of the genome of different microbes by genetic engineering methods. They have a much higher discriminatory power, which makes them suitable to use for evolution and molecular clock studies, as well as epidemiological and pathogenicity investigations. However, the technique is difficult and the cost is also high.

Three main methods have been developed to study the genetic relatedness of micro-organisms:

- by direct comparison of the DNA sequence – the number of differences between the comparative DNA sequences is related to the number of mutations, and gives information about the time of divergence
- by indirect comparison:
  - restriction fragment length polymorphism (RFLP) analysis – general method for other typing methods, based on a comparison of the fragments of DNA by their length, which correlates with the number of nucleotide substitutions after the digestion of genome by an endonuclease enzyme
  - DNA–DNA hybridization; the thermal stability of homoduplex DNA molecules (having no mismatches and thus originating from the same source) is higher than that of heteroduplex DNA molecules

(having mismatches and thus originating from different sources) by creating artificial hybrid DNA molecules.

Genotyping methods require the presence of isolates at the same time, and the results of different laboratories cannot be compared – except for reporting the complete sequence, which requires the storage of isolates.

Summary

This chapter has indicated the major causes of hospital-acquired infection, and the following points have been highlighted:

- Micro-organisms are the essential cause of infectious diseases, within the concept of the 'causal pie'.
- Bacteria, viruses and fungi are the most frequent causes of both community- and hospital-acquired infection because of their close adaptation to human conditions and worldwide occurrence.
- Most of the bacteria and fungi that cause HAI belong to the normal flora of the body, which reflects their relative pathogenicity (see Chapter 2), indicating that human endogenous risk factors are also essential elements in these infections.
- Our knowledge about the microbes causing infectious diseases is growing. For a long time it was thought that viruses containing a gene-coding substance were the smallest micro-organisms. However, infective prions do not contain nucleic acid but are still able to infect humans. It is not known whether there are lipids, polysaccharides or other substances, both organic and inorganic, that are able to cause infections, but theoretically this may happen. Prions are the newest challenge in the aetiology of diseases, which may eclipse the current problems of infection control for most resistant spore-forming bacteria, in both community and hospitals.
- The role of microbiology in the accurate diagnosis of infectious diseases has been increasing for the following reasons:
  - the appearance and discovery of new micro-organisms on the phylogenetic tree due to the process of evolution (such as HIV)
  - the discovery of pathogens causing diseases previously thought to be non-infectious (*Helicobacter pylori*, *Borrelia burgdorferi*)
  - the re-emergence of 'old' well-known pathogens in more resistant forms (methicillin-resistant *Staphylococci*, vancomycin-resistant *Enterococci*).

- Effective microbiological diagnosis begins with a decision about the method of specimen collection and its practical execution.
- The sensitivity and specificity of a laboratory test is only part of the total sensitivity and specificity of the microbiological investigation.
- Quality control of the microbiological investigation is important for the correct diagnosis of infectious disease.
- It is the responsibility of the microbiologist to provide clinicians regularly with the results of the validation of tests used in the microbiological laboratory.

Chapter 2

Infection and its characteristics

Disease versus the healthy state

A key concept of medicine is to know the natural history of disease, of both infectious and non-infectious origin. The natural history of a disease is a process that begins with exposure to the factor(s), or the accumulation of those factors, that finally cause the disease if no intervention takes place. The final outcome of exposure to the causal factor(s) depends on the relative hazard of the factor(s) to the individual, which is generally called the susceptibility of the host.

In generally, the outcome of any health-related event after exposure to any potential hazardous factor can be grouped into two broad categories:

- disease
- healthy state.

Disease, in medical terms, is a sum of the pathological changes in the tissues of a macro-organism in response to the causal factor(s), and which can be detected by macroscopic and/or microscopic pathological methods. Pathological changes may or may not be detected by strictly physical methods (visual inspection, touch), or other diagnostic methods (laboratory methods, imaging, such as X-ray, computer tomography, ultrasound).

In subjective terms, disease is the subjective feelings of the patient on recognizing and accepting the clinical signs (if they are perceptible) as a disease, in which case they are called 'complaints'. Disease is an indicator of the quality of health and the health care system.

Different causal factors may cause the same or different pathological changes leading to similar or different diseases. For example, both hepatitis B and hepatitis C can cause the same outcomes: acute or chronic hepatitis, or hepatocellular carcinoma.

A *healthy state* occurs if pathological changes do not develop in response to the exposure to a causal factor, i.e. it has no significance for the macro-organism as a potential hazard. The host does not have any subjective complaints and feels himself or herself to be healthy. However, a molecular biological reaction may occur, producing reactive factors indirectly indicating the contact. Pathological changes without clinical signs are not the same as the healthy state because they contribute to the asymptomatic form of a disease. The terms 'disease' and 'healthy state' are mutually exclusive at any point in time, i.e. they can follow each other but they cannot occur at the same time in one host.

Recovery from a disease may result in the complete disappearance of pathological changes in the tissues, but the disease may turn into disability with permanent damage to tissues leading to a decreased function of the attacked organs. The opposite of recovery is death, which is a possible outcome of severe disease. Thus, on the health scale we have the progression: *health – mild disease – severe disease – death.*

Lethality is used to express mathematically the severity of a disease; it is the proportion of deaths among those who develop the disease. The higher the lethality, the more life threatening the disease. For example, the lethality of septic shock in hospitals is above 60%. Another example is rabies, with 100% lethality.

The *'pattern of a disease'* is the natural flow of a disease. Pattern: 'A model or design, or a set of facts or conditions considered as composing an integrated design' (Churchill's, 1989, p.1397). A disease may have one or more different patterns. Generally the pattern of a disease is distinguished at two levels:

• individual level
• population level.

Variation in pathological changes leads to different clinical outcomes, giving the individual patterns or 'pictures' of a disease. Patterns of diseases at the individual level may affect the disease patterns at the population level. Describing the patterns of diseases is part of disease research. Understanding individual and population patterns of diseases is a basic element in therapeutic and preventive medicine.

In life we are exposed to different potential hazard factors: physical, chemical, biological and psychical. Biohazard in humans is caused by other biological organisms with a potential to cause disease or even death:

- macro-organisms:
  - bites, scratches:
    - wild animals (snakes, flies, ticks)
    - domestic animals (dogs, cats, etc.)
- micro-organisms – infection.

Definition of 'infection'

Infection is defined as a process in which an infectious agent is present and is able to grow and multiply in the tissues of a macro-organism. The word *infection* comes from the Latin: *inficere* = to dip in, to dye, to stain, from *in* = into + *facere* = to make, to treat, to prepare (Churchill's, 1989, p. 939).

The macro-organism, which is usually a larger organism than the infectious agent, is called the host. All infection should be regarded as a 'host–infectious agent' association. We have been exposed to infectious agents continuously since birth. Survival is genetically determined in both humans and micro-organisms in order to keep the species alive on Earth. Interaction between microbes and humans may be regarded as a 'continuous war' to survive. Infectious diseases are distinguished from non-infectious diseases in several respects:

- the causal agents are living organisms that have special life cycles
- the host can be protected against the agent
- there is a possibility of infectiousness or transmissibility of the agent from one host to another.

Infectious process in the host

An *infectious process* is the set of elements, at an individual level, which is characteristic of the infectious agents only in the case of the susceptibility of the host:

- maintenance of the infectious agent:
  - attachment to the host
  - local or general spread in the host
  - multiplication in the host
  - evasion of the host defences
  - shedding from the host (transmission)
- ability to cause disease – pathogenicity.

The elements of maintenance are essential and common to all infectious agents for the production of offspring.

Attachment to the host is the first step in the infectious process that follows exposure to an infectious agent. It is the process whereby an infectious agent connects with the host tissue cells at the portal of entry. The means of attachment can be grouped into two broad categories according to the portal of entry:

- superficial tissues:
  - skin
  - mucosa of:
    - eye
    - respiratory tract
    - urinary tract
    - genital tract
    - alimentary tract
- deep tissues:
  - insect bites
  - scratches, injury.

The common feature of tissues having direct contact with the environment is that their surfaces are covered with epithelial cells that play a role in the mechanical defence of these barriers. The epithelium of the skin is the most resistant. Secretions from the epithelial tissue (especially in mucosa) also promote defence by covering the epithelial surface, thus preventing the attachment of microbes to the epithelial cells. Successful attachment needs specific receptors at the host's epithelial tissues, and adhesins on the surface of the microbes. When a microbe is introduced into deep tissues (by bites, injury, etc.) then the attachment is made to the deep tissues directly. Four mechanisms for the development of an infection have been described (modification of categories given by Mims and colleagues) (Mims et al., 2001, p. 10):

- intact anti-microbial defences of the host:
  - active microbial attachment
- impaired anti-microbial defences in the host:
  - attachment due to mechanical injury of outer layers:
    - skin wound, mucosal injury
    - arthropod biting
    - local and general defects in the body.

Active microbial attachment occurs when the integrity of barriers (skin and mucosa) is intact and the infectious agent attaches due to its natural ability. For example, in the case of syphilis *Treponema pallidum* can attach to intact skin or the mucosa of the genital tract. Another example is leptospirosis, when the *Leptospira* species occurring in puddles or in still water may infect humans through the skin of bare feet.

Impaired anti-microbial defences help such microbes to attach that are not capable of attaching by themselves. Preliminary damage to, or impairment of, the defences decreases the resistance of the outer layers, so promoting attachment and even invasion. *Mechanical injury* of the skin or mucosa serves as a gate for the entry and attachment of an infectious agent. *Arthropod biting* helps to introduce infectious agents that could not otherwise be actively attached to the host because of the lack of a natural adhesin system. This is one of the most common mechanisms for viral infections (known as arthropod-borne infections), and malaria is a common example.

Local and general defects of the barriers and defences may promote the attachment and penetration of infectious agents even without preliminary mechanical injury. This is due to a decrease in local and general immunity, and it is a characteristic of opportunistic pathogens or facultative pathogens.

Most HAI falls into the category of impaired defences of the host due to mechanical injuries of the outer layers, or to a decrease in local and general defences.

The *local or general spreading* of an infectious agent is the second step in the infection process. In local spreading the microbe stays in the superficial tissue, where it attaches to or penetrates the subepithelial layers of the barrier tissue without invading the deep organs. If the infectious process involves organs distant from the place of attachment further spreading is necessary (see Figure 2.1). Spreading into the deep tissues of the host is known as general spreading or invasion, which may be achieved in the following ways:

- via circulating body fluids:
  - lymphatics
  - blood system
- by direct spreading.

Invading microbes inevitably reach the circulating body fluids (lymphatics and blood vessels) in the subepithelial layers. Microbes can multiply in the

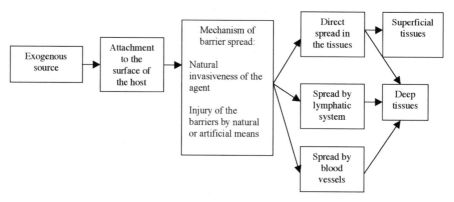

Figure 2.1. Infectious process.

lymph nodes, either remaining there or spreading in order to reach their distant organ targets. Spreading is connected with the tropism of microbes, which is defined as the affinity of microbes for specific tissue cells of the organs. The speed of spreading in lymphatic capillaries is much slower than in blood vessels (haematogenous spreading).

Direct spreading occurs if an infectious agent, resistant to local defence mechanisms, moves into the neighbouring tissues where the attachment has occurred. Toxins and enzymes produced by the micro-organisms help to destroy the connective tissues of the host, cutting a passage for the spread of the microbes. Directly spreading microbes can cause serious tissue damage, for example necrotizing fascitis caused by the toxin-producing strains of *Streptococcus pyogenes*. Pneumonia, tracheo-bronchitis or skin infections are other examples.

Multiplication is the main mechanism for the infectious agents to maintain themselves, which occurs in the most optimal tissues. Replication of microbes is different from that of humans in that thousands or millions of offspring may be produced in several hours or days. This explains the rapid adaptation of microbes to unfavourable circumstances by the selection of resistant mutants during multiplication. Mutations are responsible for the development of resistance against antibiotics and disinfectants.

The general spread and multiplication of an infectious agent may involve several stages, which are usually called primary, secondary, tertiary, etc. The stage from attachment until reaching the first multiplication location is called the primary spread and primary focus of multiplication. If an infectious agent spreads from the primary focus to another organ and multiplies there, then it is called secondary spread and secondary focus.

This is quite common for *Staphylococcus* sepsis, where the bacterium spreads from the primary focus (for example skin wound infection) into bones, causing secondary osteomyelitis.

Evading host defences is most important for enabling microbes to survive, so promoting both the spread and multiplication in the host. This is also achieved by the production of factors inhibiting the host defence mechanisms.

Shedding from the host (transmission) is a fundamental element of the infectious process, which involves leaving the host to enter the environment and hence to infect another host (see Chapter 3). Portal(s) of exit are the leaving points in the host that are the optimal places for microbes to achieve this.

Immunity and susceptibility

Interaction between microbes and a host involves the immediate reaction of the host against the microbe as 'foreign'. The development of 'immunology' as a new medical sub-science has greatly helped to understand such interaction. The word 'immune' means 'protected'; it comes from the Latin: *immunis* (*im* = not + *munus* = duty, task, service) exempt (Churchill's, 1989, p. 919). Immunology deals with the general protection of the host.

An *antigen* is a substance that is recognized by a host as being a foreign body. An antigen entering the host provokes the mobilization of the protective factors of the host. Infectious agents are also recognized by the host as foreign bodies by means of antigens – foreign molecules on the surface of the micro-organisms (polysaccharides, proteins and other molecules).

Protection against infectious agents is maintained by the three main types of immunity:

- species-related – the host is genetically resistant to the microbe, which cannot attach to and grow in or on the host's tissues
- aspecific – which reacts against every substance recognized as foreign to the host:
  - the barrier function of the skin and mucosa
  - aspecific humoral factors (acidity of stomach, saliva)
  - aspecific immune cells (natural killers, macrophages)
- specific – which reacts specifically against foreign bodies (called antigens) after recognition of the foreign body. According to the type of immunological reaction, there are two types of specific immunity:

- humoral immunity – specific humoral factors first producing immunoglobulins of class M, and then immunoglobulins of class G
- cellular immunity or cell-mediated immunity (CMI) – the proliferation of lymphotic cells of class T (thymus-dependent) leading to cellular immunity (helpers, killers and other cells).

Specific immunity can be further sub-classified according to where the immune factors produced are:

- active – when the host develops immunity internally by exposure to immunogen antigens from outside, or
- passive – immune factors are produced in an external host and are then transferred to the recipient. The immune system of the recipient is not actively involved in the production of immune factors.

Both active and passive specific immunity can be further classified (see Figure 2.2) as:

- natural – if the specific immunity is developed or acquired in a natural way without conscious human intervention

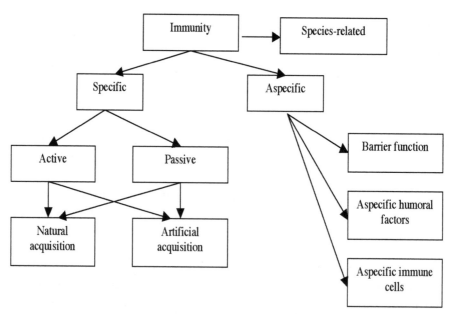

Figure 2.2. Classification of immunity.

- artificial – if the specific immunity is acquired by conscious human intervention (vaccination, immunoglobulins).

Natural active immunity is acquired if the host survives a natural infection (clinical or asymptomatic) and produces specific factors of humoral and/or cellular immunity.

Natural passive immunity occurs when the antibodies of class G penetrate from a pregnant woman through the placenta into the foetus. These antibodies may circulate and can be detected in the newborn for up to six months after birth, protecting the new baby from such infections. The foetus acquires only antibodies against those infectious agents with which the mother had been infected before or during the pregnancy, and the antibodies of which are still circulating at the time of pregnancy.

Artificial immunity, both active and passive, is achieved by immunization of the host; this is called artificial immunization.

Artificial active immunity is achieved by the antigen from the infectious agent entering the host, forcing him or her to react actively, thereby developing specific immunity. The antigen in any form is called a 'vaccine' and the process is called 'vaccination' (see Chapter 3).

Artificial passive immunity is achieved by introducing ready-made immunoglobulins (antibodies) into the body of the host by injection. If the amount of antibody introduced is adequate the host becomes immune immediately because there is no need for self-development of the immune factors (see Chapter 3).

Susceptibility is the opposite immunity. In old terminology, it meant resistance to a disease (Mims et al., 2001, p. 361). But in modern medical terminology it has a wider meaning: 'susceptible: Liable to infection or to the effects of substances, as toxins or other influences; lacking the capacity to respond effectively to a pathogen'. It has a Latin origin: *suscipere* = to lift up, undergo + *ible* English meaning: capable of undergoing (Churchill's, 1989, p. 1827).

In the concept of infection: susceptible: 'A person or animal not possessing sufficient resistance against a particular pathogenic agent to prevent contracting infection or disease when exposed to the agent' (Chin, 2000, p. 578).

Perfect resistance against infectious agents is attained by species-related immunity, while the other mechanisms of immunity (aspecific and specific) may not be able to resist the infection completely. Currently we distinguish 'susceptibility to an infection' from 'susceptibility to a disease' because they are two levels on the susceptibility scale. Others explain this as the independence of these two forms of susceptibility (Mims et al., 2001, p. 361):

- susceptibility to infection – the possibility of the agent to attach to and grow in, or on, the host
- susceptibility to disease – the host's reaction to the infection by the development of disease against the attached and growing agent.

There is evidence that three factors have a substantial influence on the outcome of an infection:

- the initial dose of an infectious agent per single case of infection
- the immunity level of the host
- the ability of the agent to cause disease (pathogenicity or virulence).

The *infecting dose* is defined as the number of viable particles of an infectious agent per single infection episode. By convention – taken from experimental disease research and toxicology – such a minimal dose of an agent is defined as that which produces the expected effect in 50% of those inoculated (D_{50}). Three types of infecting dose have been developed for infections:

- infectious dose (ID_{50})
- disease-producing dose (DD_{50})
- lethal dose (LD_{50}).

ID_{50} expresses the susceptibility to the infection, showing the necessary minimal viable quantity of the agent to cause effective infection in 50% of cases. It is not necessary that individuals will develop disease after acquiring such a dose.

DD_{50} characterizes the minimal dose required to cause disease, while LD_{50} is the dose needed to cause death in 50% of those who have been exposed to the agent.

In practice we do not know precisely the infecting dose per case, but it can be estimated from data obtained from experiments on human, animals or tissue cultures (Mims et al., 2001, p. 362). For example, only ten viable cells of *Shigella dysenteriae* are enough to cause clinical dysentery in 50% of exposed persons (Mims et al., 2001, p. 362). If someone develops dysentery then we assume that the infecting dose has reached the disease-producing dose (DD) of ten viable cells of the agent.

Obviously the higher the infecting dose per single infectious episode the higher the probability that the infection will result in disease or death.

Immunity level against micro-organisms is not stable in individuals as it may change over time in both directions as a result of several factors, for example, reinfection, ageing, gender, nutritional state or underlying diseases – especially diseases of the immune system. A decrease of the immune function for any reason may lead to a smaller dose being required to cause infection, or disease with a lethal outcome.

Wane of immunity occurs if a person who has been immunized by natural or artificial means again becomes susceptible to the infection because the immune factors drop below the level offering protection. However, being infected again may lead to a milder form of disease than the first time due to residual immunity known as 'immune memory'. An example is whooping cough among elderly people who survived the infection in their childhood.

The function of the immune system in an individual can be determined by two main methods:

- laboratory methods
- modelling.

Laboratory methods aim to measure quantitatively and qualitatively the function of both aspecific and specific immune systems to discover any deficiency in their function. Laboratory methods have several applications, with diagnostic and screening purposes:

- to diagnose primary disorders of the immune system, both congenital and acquired forms
- checking antibody levels against a specific microbe
- to confirm immunodeficiency because of underlying diseases, e.g. diabetes.

In advanced disease research, *modelling* has been developed to understand and to separate the patterns of an infection by classifying them according to different models (Anderson and May, 1991; Mollison, 1995). For an individual, different categories of immunity define the host–infectious agent association:

- susceptible (S)
- infected (I):

  – without disease: colonized or carrier (C)
  – diseased (D)
- recovered:
  – has become immune or resistant (R)
  – remains susceptible (S).

In individual models of an infection, these categories describe what is happening with an individual in the infection process. Persistence of an infectious agent is the form of infected state when the host is not able to get rid of the infectious agent.

'Catalytic' models have been developed to describe the patterns according to the immunity and persistence of the infection (Muench 1959; Hillis 1979; Zhang 1987).

A *simple catalytic model* describes the infectious process when the susceptible host becomes infected and remains so for his or her life, without the clearance of the infectious agent from the body because of an ineffective immune system – SI. If the agent survives on the surface of the host it is called 'colonization', which is mainly a feature of bacteria and fungi. If the agent lives inside the body of the host it is usually called the 'carrier' stage. For many viral and protozoal infections it is a method of survival (e.g. hepatitis B and C, HIV, toxoplasma) (see Figure 2.3).

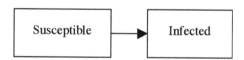

Figure 2.3. Simple catalytic model of an infection.

A *reversible catalytic model* is where a host who is susceptible (S) becomes infected (I) and then reverts to the stage of susceptibility after the infection is self-limited or cured by medical intervention – SIS (Figure 2.4). This happens in tetanus, where the natural infection does not lead to immunity (WHO, 1996). Another example is influenza, when a host surviving the infection loses the specific immunity after several years and again becomes

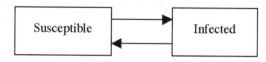

Figure 2.4. Reversible catalytic model of an infection.

susceptible. Whooping cough occurs quite often in elderly people after infection in childhood, but in a milder form.

A *two-stage catalytic model* occurs if a susceptible (S) host is infected (I) and becomes resistant (R) against an infectious agent for the whole lifetime – SIR. This is the basis of lifelong immunity. It is believed that many viral infections (for example, measles, rubella) fall into this category (see Figure 2.5).

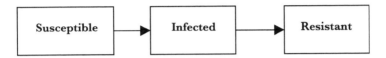

Figure 2.5. Two-stage catalytic model of an infection.

Parasitism and pathogenicity

Any organism needs nutritional factors for reproduction, to maintain its structure and other life needs. Biological organisms usually do not live alone – they interact with each other in the environment. This interaction is called a biological association, and may take one of four forms:

• parasitic
• symbiotic
• commensalism
• indifference.

Parasitic association is where one organism benefits at the expense of another. The best example is the so-called intracellular micro-organisms that can live and replicate only in the cells of another host (for example, viruses, rickettsia, gonococcus). Living in a host cell will usually lead to the death or other destruction of the host cells, causing damage to the host tissues and organs.

Symbiotic association occurs when both organisms benefit. For humans this form is less obvious, and the most recent data have shown that microbes comprising the human flora thought to be harmless may cause diseases if the host's defences are decreased. For example, the role of *Staphylococcus epidermidis* of the skin flora has been demonstrated in infections associated with implants (Dickinson and Bisno, 1989a, 1989b). Another example is the *Corynebacterium* species causing meningitis after lumbar puncture. However, *Lactobacillus*, which increases the acidity in the vagina, contributes to the defence mechanism in women.

Commensalism is where one organism benefits without causing damage to another. This is an intermediate form between the symbiotic and parasitic forms. It is difficult to define this form because detailed examination will prove that the association is either symbiotic or parasitic.

Indifference occurs if the two organisms receive no benefit or harm if they are in contact.

In medicine a term similar to parasitism is 'pathogenicity', which is used to describe the biological association between a human and another biological organism – usually a micro-organism. The infectious agent causing an infectious disease is called a *pathogen* and the process is *pathogenicity*. *Pathogen* is of Greek origin: *patho* = *paschein* = to undergo, to be affected + *gen* = *gennan* = to beget, to produce, to create (Churchill's, 1989, p. 775). The pathogenicity of a micro-organism is always relative to the host, and it should be evaluated for each specific host. The pathogenicity of microbes towards humans can be divided into four main categories; however, there are no fixed borders between the categories:

- absolute pathogens
- facultative pathogens
- opportunistic pathogens
- non-pathogens.

An *absolute* pathogen causes disease in any circumstances when the host is exposed to it. An example is anthrax caused by *Bacillus anthracis* – a very dangerous pathogen with a fatal outcome.

Facultative pathogens cause diseases only in specific and appropriate conditions. Pathogenicity of microbes of this group is strongly associated with the *lack* of defence mechanisms in the host. For example, *Escherichia coli*, an inhabitant of the gut with no disease, may cause urinary tract infection, wound infection, brain abscess or even blood poisoning. However, some strains of *Escherichia coli* may also produce toxins causing disease of the gut (diarrhoea by enteropathogen *Escherichia coli*) or other organs (e.g. kidney) (see Chapter 6).

Opportunistic pathogens are those causing disease only in an immunocompromized host with defective humoral and/or cell-mediated immunity. Among them, *Pneumocystis carinii* is the most frequent in patients with acquired immune deficiency syndrome (AIDS).

Non-pathogens do not cause disease in any circumstances because the germ is indifferent to the host, or symbiotic association occurs. This is called zero pathogenicity (Mims et al., 2001).

Most human infections are caused by facultative pathogen microbes with medium pathogenicity, which is explained by the concept of 'balanced pathogenicity' (Mims et al., 2001, p. 4). If all the infectious agents were absolute parasites, they would kill all the hosts, which would terminate their existence as well, because there would be no host to accommodate them. The more usual pattern is, for example, sexually transmitted diseases caused by various microbes (*Neisseria gonorrhoeae*, *Treponema pallidum*, *Human herpes virus*, *Trichomonas vaginalis*, etc.), which cause mild diseases without killing the human host, thus ensuring that they can maintain themselves, and replicate.

A term closely related to 'pathogenicity' is 'virulence': 'The pathogenicity or disease-producing capacity of any infectious agent' (Churchill's, 1989, p. 2086). However, there are measures to express pathogenicity and virulence separately: pathogenicity refers to the proportion of infected people who develop the disease, while virulence refers to the proportion of severely ill patients or deaths among those who become ill (US Department of Health and Human Services, 1992, p. 44). Thus pathogenicity is a broader term than virulence. Sometimes it is difficult to establish the border between mild and severe disease, and so the lethality is the best measure of virulence.

Pathogenicity and virulence may vary among strains of the same microbe, which result in different clinical outcomes if persons are infected with strains of different pathogenicity and virulence (Greene, 1996).

Inapparent and clinical infection

According to pathogenicity, for practical infection control the final outcome of an infection in humans is usually divided into two well-distinguishable forms:

- manifest (clinical) infection
- inapparent (asymptomatic) infection.

Manifest (clinical) infection is the result of the interaction between microbial and reacting host factors, leading to pathological changes. It develops if the virulence factors of the infectious agent overwhelm the resistance factors of the host. Clinical infection (infectious disease) shows general (aspecific) signs of the disease (fever, fatigue, seizure, etc.) and/or specific signs characteristic of the specific infectious disease (e.g. type of rash in measles, or watery diarrhoea in cholera, etc.). Clinical signs are used for the differential diagnosis of infectious diseases with clinical importance. However, they are of paramount importance for *case definition*, including HAI, in public health in general (see Chapter 4).

The flow of an infectious disease in an individual is the result of the infectious process within the host, which has well-defined consecutive moments and phases (see Figure 2.6):

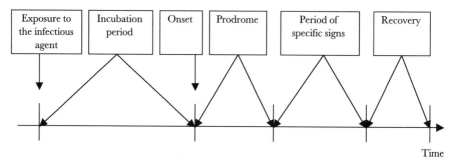

Figure 2.6. Phases of the infectious process in a host with manifest infection.

- exposure to the infectious agent
- incubation period
- onset of the disease
- prodrome
- period of manifest clinical signs
- recovery/disability/death.

Exposure to the infectious agent is the moment when the host contacts the infectious agent and the agent attaches to the host.

The incubation period is defined as the time from exposure to the infectious agent until the onset of the first (not necessarily the first specific) clinical sign. This time is needed for the infectious agent to grow and to cause a reaction from the host by developing pathological changes. The word 'incubation' is of Latin origin: *incubare* = to lie or sit on, brood, from *in-* = in, on + *cubare* = to lie (Churchill's, 1989, p. 933). This period is characteristic of each infectious agent, and it has a range with minimum and maximum values (Chin, 2000). The incubation period serves to define the possible date of the exposure of the host to an infectious agent:

- the minimum incubation period – the latest date of the exposure
- the maximum value – the earliest date of the exposure.

This is important for defining the day of exposure, which serves to distinguish infection imported to a hospital from hospital-acquired infection.

Onset is the moment when the first clinical sign appears. The date, and even the time of the beginning of clinical signs, can be provided by the patient.

Prodome is characterized by the presence of early clinical signs that may be common for different infectious agents without any specificity (general prodrome), but in some infections it is quite specific and the type of the infectious agent can be identified by this (specific prodrome). The word 'prodrome' is Greek in origin: *pro-* = before, ahead + *dromos* = a race, running (Churchill's, 1989, p. 1524).

The period of manifest signs is when the clinical signs that are usually characteristic of a given infectious agent are present. It originates from the word 'manifestation', which comes from the Latin: *manifestare* = to make evident, make clear, from *manus* = the hand + *-festus* = as *in-festus* = hostile, aggressive (Churchill's, 1989, p. 1101).

Recovery phase refers to the disappearance of clinical signs, and the restoration of health and strength. This phase is also called convalescence. If the outcome is severe, the death of the patient may occur instead of recovery. Disability may occur, with permanent functional damage to the affected organs.

A clinical infection may last for several days or for the rest of an individual's life, depending on the different pattern of each infection. Two types of manifest infection are distinguished, according to their duration:

- acute manifest infection
- chronic manifest infection.

An *acute manifest infection* has a definite end to the clinical signs, usually within three months after the start of the illness, which distinguishes it from chronic disease (Last, 1995, p. 28). The word 'acute' comes from Latin: *acuere* = to sharpen, incite, stimulate, characterized by sudden onset, marked symptoms, and a short course: said especially of a disease (Churchill's, 1989, p. 24). There are two main subtypes according to the 'flow' of the disease:

- typical
- atypical.

The 'flow' of clinical infection is typical if all the specific clinical signs characteristic of the infection are present.

In atypical 'flow', the specific signs are not all present, only general signs, which makes it difficult to categorize the disease.

A *chronic manifest infection* is of longer duration than the acute. In the USA it is defined as three months or longer (Last, 1995, p. 28). It may cause disability in the patient and result in higher cost to both the patient and society due to the continuing flow of the infection and the accumulation of such patients. In hospitals, chronic HAI (for example chronic osteomyelitis) contributes to longer stays in hospitals and increased health care costs, which is a logical reason to control and prevent HAI (Haley et al., 1980c).

Inapparent (*asymptomatic*) infection occurs if no recognizable clinical signs are present during the growth of the infectious agent within the host. This is due to the balance between the virulence of the microbe and the resistance factors of the host against the microbe.

The term 'infection' is not synonymous with the term 'infectious disease' (Last, 1995, p. 85). Last's distinction will be used throughout this book and it will be made clear if the subtype of the infection has any special feature. If not, then both types (manifest and inapparent) are to be understood by the term 'infection'.

Because an inapparent infection has no clinical signs, the periods of the infectious process – defined for manifest infection – have no meaning for this type of infection. However, the essential steps of the infectious process for the maintenance of an infectious agent (attachment, spread, multiplication, shedding) can be established.

Both manifest and inapparent infection can be independent outcomes of an infectious process, or they can be in strong relation, being successive phases of the same infectious process.

Recurrent clinical infection occurs if an inapparent infection becomes manifest, usually as a result of a decrease in the defence mechanism of the host. This process is called exacerbation. A good example is the recurrent herpes caused by the herpes simplex virus. Many recurrent infections (e.g. toxoplasma, herpes, cytomegalovirus) occur among individuals with acquired immunodeficiency syndrome, which confirms the need for a 'perfect' immune system to prevent exacerbation of persisting inapparent infections.

Period of infectiousness

The *period of infectiousness* is that period during which the host is able to spread an infectious agent into the environment after harbouring the agent on the surface of the body or in the deep tissues. For many infections the period of infectiousness is well defined, for example chicken pox, measles

(Chin, 2000). However, for many infections with an inapparent or chronic pattern the duration of the colonization or carrier stage can be undefined, and it may last for several days or years, or even for the rest of the individual's life. For example, a certain proportion of the patients may carry *Salmonella typhi* for life after recovering from typhoid fever. The period of infectiousness depends on the ability of the immune system to clear an infectious agent from the body of the host. A synonym is 'period of communicability' (Chin, 2000, p. 560).

Complex patterns of infections

Manifest or inapparent infections and their duration may produce even more complex patterns of infection if combined with the development of immunity and clearance of the microbe. Figure 2.7 illustrates the stages and the possible outcomes if a susceptible host is infected.

The first stage of an infection entails one of the alternative clinical outcomes: inapparent infection or disease. In the second stage, if immunity is quite strong, the host is cleared of the infectious agent and may remain immune for life, or may become susceptible again due to wane of immunity. If immunity is not strong enough to clear the infection the host remains infected inapparently, or chronic infection develops. Remission of clinical signs of a chronic infection, i.e. disappearance of pathological changes, also depends on the immunity. Several patterns of infection can be drawn when a host moves from one stage to another. An infectious agent may have several patterns, which reflects the variation of the microbe–host interaction. This is illustrated in the example of the hepatitis B infection (see Figure 2.8).

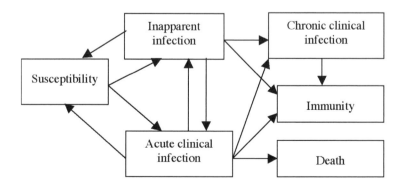

Figure 2.7. Flow patterns of infection in a susceptible host.

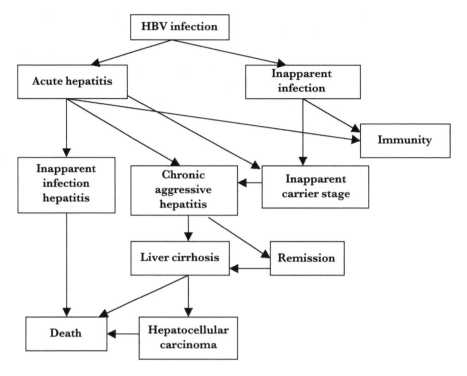

Figure 2.8. Patterns of hepatitis B (HBV) infection.

Summary

This chapter summarizes the essential characteristics of an infection in a host. The following points are the most important:

- The infectious process describes the flow of an infection at the individual level, while the dynamics of an infection are at the population level (see Chapter 3).
- Virulence is the internal ability of a microbe to cause disease, while pathogenicity is the net result of the virulence and host's defence system.
- The term 'infection' relates to both inapparent and clinical infection.
- Any outcome of an infection depends on the susceptibility of the host. Complete immunity prevents even the attachment of an infectious agent, while incomplete immunity may prevent a serious outcome, but it is not able to prevent the agent from attaching to and growing in the host. There is a tendency to call incomplete immunity 'partial immunity'.

- The infectious process does not differ in community-acquired infection (CAI) from hospital-acquired infection (HAI).
- The concept of dose-dependence has been accepted to estimate the outcome of an infection. It is also the basis of a preventive strategy regarding infections in both the community and hospitals, reducing the dose of microbial contact by decontamination (see Chapter 5).

CHAPTER 3

The chain of infection and the transmission of an infective agent

Infections from an external source – the chain of infection

The chain of infection is defined as the transmission of an infectious agent from one habitation to another (see Figure 3.1). Three loops are involved in the transmission: reservoir (source) of the infection – mode of transmission – susceptible host. Transmissibility is the fundamental property of infectious agents.

The concept of transmission is the basic principle of infection control because by interrupting the transmission at any stage we can prevent the spread of an infectious agent in the environment, thus preventing the occurrence of new infected cases. This is achieved by:

- finding and eliminating the reservoir or source
- finding and eliminating the mode of transmission
- protecting the portals of entry or making the recipient host resistant to the infectious agent and preventing the further growth and multiplication of the infectious agent in the host.

These are general principles and can be applied to both HAI and community-acquired infection (CAI).

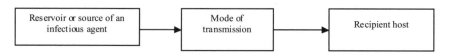

Figure 3.1. Chain of infection.

Reservoir of infection

The *reservoir* (source) of the infectious agent is the habitat (man, animals, plants, inanimate environment) where the infectious agent lives, grows and multiplies, depending primarily for survival in such a manner that it can be transmitted to another habitat (Top, 1967 p. 65). 'Reservoir' is of French origin: from *réserver* = to reserve, from the Latin *reservare* = to lay up, keep back.

Infections can be classified according to their main reservoirs:

* anthroponosis – man is the only reservoir (e.g. typhoid fever caused by *Salmonella typhi*)
* zoonosis – animals are only the reservoir and humans are not a reservoir of the infectious agent (e.g. trichinellosis caused by *Trichinella spiralis*)
* zoo-anthroponosis – the main reservoir is animals, and humans can be infected by transmission of the infectious agent from the animals or additionally from another human (e.g. salmonellosis-caused *Salmonella* species, influenza).

The transmission of an infectious agent from the reservoir is characterized by two features:

* mode of transmission;
* reproduction (transmissibility) measures.

Modes of transmission of infectious agents

Mode of transmission is defined as the way in which an infectious agent spreads from the source into the environment. When the reservoir of an infectious agent is man or animals then the *sites* of the localization of the infection, from where the agent can be transmitted, define the portal of exit determining the mode(s) of transmission of the infectious agent into the environment. For humans the following sites play a role in transmission:

* sites having direct contact with the outside world:
  – skin
  – mucous membranes of:
    ○ respiratory tract

- ○ gastrointestinal tract
- ○ genitourinary tract
- ○ eye
- sites not having direct contact with the outside world:
  - – bloodstream
  - – deep tissues.

Those infectious agents at the sites that do not have direct contact with the outside world can leave the host only after an interruption of barrier tissues.

Transmission can be effective only if the links of the chain are contiguous via the contact. Knowledge of the mechanism of the contact between the links is important when drawing up the chain of infection. Mechanisms of contact can be:

- direct contact between the reservoir (source) and the recipient host:
  - – human-to-human:
    - ○ droplets – sneezing, coughing, talking
    - ○ direct physical:
      - ▫ kissing – social behaviour, sexual practices
      - ▫ skin-to-skin – touch, hand-shaking, patient care
      - ▫ mucosa-to-mucosa – sexual intercourse
      - ▫ faecal–oral – hand, sexual practices
    - ○ skin squama
  - – soil-to-person – agriculture, cooking
  - – vegetation-to-person – agriculture, cooking
  - – animal-to-human – bites
- indirect contact between the reservoir and the recipient host:
  - – vehicle-borne (inanimate):
    - ○ air – droplet nuclei, dust, skin squama
    - ○ comestibles – food, water, milk, etc.
    - ○ objects – equipment (medical instruments), dishes, toys, bedding, handkerchiefs, etc.
    - ○ biological products – blood, blood products, transplant organs, etc.
  - – vehicle-borne (animate) (= vector-borne) – mosquitoes, fleas, ticks, lice, flies:
    - ○ mechanical transmission
    - ○ biological.

Direct contact – the reservoir and the recipient host must be in close physical contact with each other, i.e. they have to be in the same place at the same time.

Indirect contact – the recipient does not encounter the reservoir direct but only via a *vehicle* harbouring the infectious agent, which links the reservoir and the recipient host.

It is important to be clear about the terms 'reservoir of infection' and 'source of infection'. In this regard, two points of view may be found in public health practice:

- According to US public health opinion, the reservoir may or may not be the source of infection. The reservoir should be distinguished from the source, which is a thing, person, object or substance from which the infectious agent passes immediately to a host (Top, 1967, p. 65). When the transmission of an infectious agent is direct from the reservoir to a habitant then the reservoir is equal to the source of infectious agent. If the transmission is indirect then the source of infection is not equal to the reservoir, but is combined with the mode of the transmission. 'For example the reservoir of *Clostridium botulinum* is soil, but the source of most botulism infections is improperly canned food containing *C. botulinum* spores' (US Department of Health and Human Services, 1992). A source of infection may contaminate other substances, which then become secondary or tertiary sources of the infection.
- In other schools of public health, like Hungary, the term 'source of infection' is equivalent to the term 'reservoir of infection' for both direct and indirect transmission of infectious agents, and the only difference is that the permanent source of the infections is generally called the reservoir. The term 'mode of transmission' is used to express the way in which an infectious agent is passed to a susceptible host, thus being a clearly separated intermediate step between the source (reservoir) of the infection and the susceptible host. Thus the triple step 'source–mode of transmission–recipient host' is always clear. For example, the reservoir (permanent source) of *Clostridium botulinum* is soil, but the mode of transmission (vehicle) of most botulism infections is improperly canned food containing *C. botulinum* spores and the source is the food factory where the food (containing spores) was prepared. These differences should be taken into account among professionals internationally because misunderstanding may happen when comparing publications from different countries.

The mode of transmission depends on the ability of the infectious agent to survive in the inanimate environment. Those that cannot survive for long are transmitted by direct means when the infectious agent passes immediately from the reservoir to the recipient host without being present in the inanimate environment (for example, *Neisseria meningitidis*, *Streptococcus pyogenes*, or sexually transmitted diseases, etc.). Those that can survive in the inanimate environment for some time can be transmitted indirectly, which is the result of adaptation to the environment (for example, *Salmonella* species).

Droplets are relatively large short-range aerosols of more than 5μ (microns) leaving the airways during physiological processes (talking, coughing, sneezing). Droplet particles contain microbes and other substances from the airways and are sprayed over a few feet, meeting the recipient before falling to the ground. Respiratory diseases are transmitted by this means, and other agents such as *Streptococcus* may also be spread in this way.

During *direct physical contact* the reservoir and the recipient are contiguous, providing the route by which the infectious particles are transmitted. Hand shaking, other forms of touching, kissing and sexual practices are the most common ways in social behaviour. In medicine, patient care and the physical examination of the patients fall into this category, and this is an important factor for HAIs.

Other types of direct contact – soil-to-human, vegetation-to-human, animal-to-human – are common in community (*Rabies, Clostridium botulinum, Echinococcus species*, etc.) but these modes of transmission do not have importance for HAIs.

Vehicle-borne is the common name for those infections when *something* transmits the infectious agent from the reservoir to a recipient host. Vehicles may passively transmit the infectious agent, or provide an environment where the agent grows, multiplies or produces toxins, which is the result of adaptation of the infectious agent to the environment, and is transmitted actively.

Droplet nuclei are the residue of dried droplets of less than 5 μ spreading from the airways by talking, sneezing or coughing but they remain in the air for a long time and may spread for a relatively long distance – up to hundreds of metres (*Variola virus, Mycobacterium tuberculosis*, etc.). They may play a role in hospitals as well.

Dust includes infectious agents from the soil and those particles that settle on to the surface of the dust from the air by re-suspension. The most common are the spore-producing microbes (*Clostridium perfringens, Bacillus anthracis*) and *Mycobacteria*. This transmission also occurs in hospitals.

Skin squama is the exfoliating cells of the skin harbouring different infectious agents, and among them *Staphylococcus* species and *Streptococcus pyogenes* are the most common. Exfoliation is a continuous process leading to the permanent spread of infectious agents by squama into the environment. Because of the epidemics of *Staphylococcus aureus* in the 1950s and 1960s British and American investigators performed a number of detailed microbiological studies to demonstrate how carriers could transmit *Staphylococcus aureus* (Rammelkamp et al., 1964; Bethune et al., 1965; Williams, 1966). These studies are classic and fundamental papers on the transmission of *Staphylococcus aureus*. Both nasal and perianal carriers continually shed staphylococci on skin squamae that serve as rafts (aptly named by British investigators) into the air. *Staphylococci* dispersed into the environment are quickly diluted by air and washed away by standard housekeeping practices. The classic study of Rammelkamp and colleagues demonstrated the spread of *Staphylococcus aureus* by the hands of staff (Rammelkamp et al., 1964).

Comestibles – food, water, milk, etc. – are those things that are used for nutrition. Food is an excellent medium for growth and toxin production. Food-poisonings are special types of infectious disease caused by toxins accumulated in the food after a period of external incubation (e.g. enterotoxins of *Staphylococcus aureus*). As nutrition is an everyday physiological need of humans, comestibles may harbour everyday hazards for those both in the community and in hospitals unless they are under strict control.

Objects contaminated by many fluids and substances can transmit different infectious agents passively. Reused medical instruments are the most dangerous objects in the transmission of infectious agents in hospitals. In the community, shared syringes and needles are common among intravenous drug users, transmitting blood-borne pathogens (HIV, hepatitis B, etc.).

Biological products are those substances that are produced by the biochemical and medical industries from tissues or cells of living organisms for agriculture, for animal husbandry and for other human purposes. The main causes of contaminated biological products are inadequate screening for the presence of infectious agents, or the agents surviving in the biological products because of ineffective decontamination. 'Mad-cow disease' is an excellent example where a series of successive transmissions has led to the development of modified Creutzfeld-Jakob disease (CJD) in humans (Brown et al., 2001). The main groups of biological products are:

- blood and blood products – plasma factors, albumin, plasma-derived vaccines, etc.

- organ transplants – kidney, heart, lungs
- tissue transplants – cornea, skin, sperm
- products of bio-fermentation – vaccines, antibiotics, other drugs, livestock.

Vector-borne infections are those in which the agent is transmitted by an insect. It can be purely mechanical transmission without biological changes of the infectious agent in the vector (such as *Shigella dysenteriae* carried by flies), or biological transmission if the agent undergoes part of its life cycle in the vector (for example *Plasmodium* species transmitted by mosquitoes). In biological transmission the vector serves as both an intermediate host and mode of transmission at the same time. The vectors are quite specific to the different infectious agents, and the occurrence of such infections depends on the presence and activity of vectors, which may vary in different climatic zones. In HAIs their roles are limited and may have importance only in those areas where the infection is commonly associated with poor hygiene.

When a human or animal is the reservoir, the infectious agent exits the reservoir at the portal exit and enters the recipient through the portal entry. As mentioned above, the portals of exit and entry determine the mode of transmission. The portal of exit corresponds to the site of localization of infection. From one portal exit the agent may be transmitted by *different* modes of transmission: for example *Shigella dysenteriae* can be transmitted directly by hand or by indirectly via food or water that has been contaminated with faeces or by flies passively (Chin, 2000). The same agent may have different localization with corresponding portals of exit, resulting in more complex alternative modes of transmission. For example, when the *Yersinia pestis* (which causes plague) is located in blood vessels of the skin it can be transmitted by fleas, but when located in the lungs of humans it is transmitted by droplet nuclei (Chin, 2000). The same agent from one portal exit may enter a different portal entry. For example, *Staphylococcus aureus* from the skin may cause skin disease in another host by the direct contact, or via equipment (e.g. medical), or it may be spread to food by hand contact and grow in the food, leading to food-poisoning (Chin, 2000). Localization of the infectious agent defines the route of transmission, which is usually named after the sites of exit and entry or after the localization of the infection. The terminology of this aspect is not complete. Table 3.1 summarizes the main categories in order to illustrate the complexity of the transmissions. For control measures it is important to know all the possible ways in which an agent can exit and enter a host (Chin, 2000).

Table 3.1. Summary of the mode of transmission of an infectious agent from the human reservoir

Route of transmission	Localization of the infectious agent	Portal of exit	Portal of entry	Mode of the transmission					
				Direct	Indirect				
					Inanimate vehicle		Comestible	Biological products	Vectors
					Air	Objects			
Faecal – oral	Gut	Gut	Mouth	Hand		Dishes, toys	Food, water		Flies
Respiratory	Airways	Airways	Airways	Droplet spread	Droplet nuclei, dust	Medical instruments			
Sexually transmitted	Genito-urinary tract	Genitals Urinary tract	Genitals Urinary tract Mucosa of other sites	Sexual intercourse		Medical instruments, towels, etc.			
Blood-borne	Bloodstream, deep tissues	Injured barriers (skin, mucosa, blood vessels)	Injured barriers (skin, mucosa, blood vessels)	Sexual intercourse		Medical instruments		Blood, blood-products, organ transplants	Fleas, lice, mosquitoes, ticks, flies
Mucosal	Mucosa of eyes	Eyes	Eyes	Hand		Towels, medical instruments, etc.		Cornea transplantation	
NS	Skin of the hand	Skin	Mouth	Hand	Skin squama	Towels, bedding, clothes, etc.	Food		
	Skin other than hand	Skin	Skin	Hand, skin squama, sexual intercourse	Skin squama				

NS = not specified.

Types of transmission between two hosts

Generally two main types of transmission can be distinguished:

- one-way transmission
- cross-transmission.

Transmission is called one-way when the reservoir harbouring a certain infectious agent spreads this agent to another host that does not harbour it (see Figure 3.2).

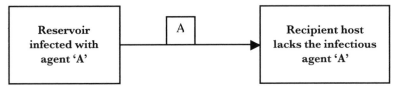

Figure 3.2. One-way transmission of infectious agent.

However, during direct contact the two hosts (in the case of human-to-human) are involved in such a way that each host may transmit its own infectious agent to the other, being a reservoir and recipient host at the same time. This called cross-transmission (Figure 3.3). For example, during

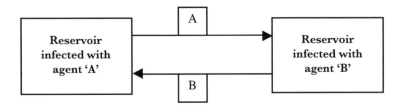

Figure 3.3. Cross-transmission of infectious agents between two different sources.

sexual intercourse an HIV-infected person may pass HIV to the sexual partner, who may harbour *Neisseria gonorrhoeae* and thus may transfer it to the HIV-infected person. Another example is when a nurse infected with *Pseudomonas aeruginosa* may spread it to patients, while she may acquire MRSA from MRSA-infected patients during patient care.

Types of transmission in a population

The appropriate connection of the three loops of the chain of infection is the elementary unit of the transmission of an infectious agent. An infectious source may transmit the agent to several recipient hosts who may then transmit the agent to other host(s) leading to *series* of chains of infection at the population level. Furthermore, transmission from one source may not be restricted to one point in time, and may be intermittent or continuous. This results in *population types* of transmission:

- common source:
  - point source
  - intermittent
  - continuous
- propagated
- mixed
- other types.

Common source means that a group of recipient hosts has been in contact with the same source. In point source transmission all hosts are in contact with the source at one point in time or within a very short period (a few hours) and those hosts who become ill will develop the disease within a minimum and maximum incubation period (see Figure 3.4).

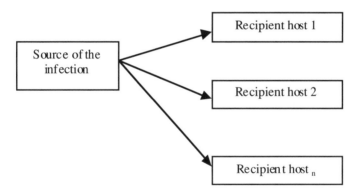

Figure 3.4. Common source of an infection.

A source may spread an infectious agent over a period in time intermittently or continuously (days, weeks, months or even years), which is a characteristic of chronic infections without the infectious agent being eliminated from the host (see Figure 3.5).

Propagated transmission occurs when an infectious agent spreads gradually from one host to another one (see Figure 3.6). The time between the appearance of the same clinical signs in the new cases is called the *serial interval*, which is important in distinguishing a common source transmission from a propagated one.

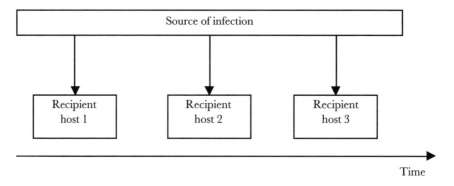

Figure 3.5. Intermittent spread of an infectious agent.

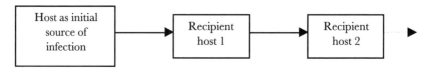

Figure 3.6. Propagated transmission of an infectious agent.

Mixed spread is the combination of common and propagated transmissions (see Figure 3.7).

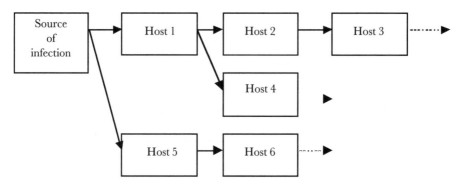

Figure 3.7. Mixed transmission of an infectious agent.

Reproduction (transmissibility) measures

In medical terms, susceptibility means that the agent can attach to, grow and multiply in the host. Successful transmission requires that the recipient host has contact with the source of the infection and is susceptible to the particular agent. If the recipient host is resistant to the agent, contact with the source will not result in transmission. However, even if the host is susceptible, not every contact with a source of an infectious agent will result in successful transmission. The effectiveness of transmission among humans can be measured both on a scale of measures between two hosts (within one chain of infection) and at the population level (serial transmission chains).

The measure of transmission between two hosts

Effective transmission of an infectious agent by a single contact between two hosts is characterized by the coefficient of the transmission.

The coefficient of transmission (β) of an infectious agent is the probability of effective transmission given a contact between the source of the infection and the susceptible recipient host. If the coefficient is equal to one it means that the transmission is 100% effective, thus the infection is unavoidable. If it is less than one it means that not every contact will result in effective transmission. If it is equal to zero the given contact will not result in transmission. For each infection it can be estimated experimentally. The coefficient of transmission is the mathematical estimate of the 'infectiousness' of an infectious agent, and concerns the relative ease with which the agent is transmitted to another susceptible host (Last, 1995, p. 85). It can be estimated by the proportion of susceptible persons exposed to the infectious agent who become infected after a specific type of contact. This coefficient is different for different contact patterns of an infectious agent, or for the same contact pattern for different infections. It is used for two purposes:

- It estimates the individual risk of being infected if a susceptible person contacts the source of infection. For example, for hepatitis B this risk is zero when the contact occurs directly with intact skin.
- It is used for the estimation of different measures of transmission at the population level.

Measures of transmission at the population level

The occurrence of an infection in a population reflects the *successful* transmissions generated by series of transmission chains. However, not every successful transmission is seen, owing to the inapparent outcome. In everyday practice the absolute measure of transmission in a population must be taken to be the number of new infected cases, regardless of the clinical outcome of the infection. Clinical cases can be found more easily than inapparent ones, which need further detection by microbiological screening. The higher the proportion of inapparent cases among the infected cases the greater the underestimation of the transmission if it relies only on clinical cases.

The transmissibility of an infectious agent in a human population depends on the following parameters:

- the characteristic of the infectious agent:
  - whether a human is the principal host
  - the infectiousness of the infectious agent at a single contact
  - the latent period
  - the duration of the infectiousness of the source
- the environmental factors:
  - the number and type of the contacts between the sources and susceptible recipient hosts
  - the frequency of the susceptible recipient hosts in the population.

As mentioned above, susceptibility is one of the requirements for effective transmission. A further condition is that the host should transmit the agent to another host. Two types of host are distinguished according to the transmission theory:

- principal host
- accidental host.

Principal host is where the infected host may serve as the further source of the infection. Anthroponotic infections occurring in humans are important, especially in hospitals, where contact between humans is the most important means of transmission of infectious agents.

An *accidental host*, while being infected, is unable to transmit the infectious agent. In this case an infected human does not play a role in the transmission. For example, a human may be an accidental host of some zoonotic infections, such as trichinellosis or rabies, but cannot transmit the infectious agent.

The *latent period* is the period from the moment of being infected until a principal host is able to transmit an infectious agent into the environment.

The *duration of infectiousness* (D) is the period of time during which a source (reservoir) remains infected and is able to transmit the agent. A synonym is 'period of communicability' (Chin, 2000). It may last for several hours, days, weeks, months or even years. It determines the possibility of intermittent or continuous spread of the agent from a source into the environment during this period. It can be estimated by following up the sources through regular microbiological screening. People who are lifelong carriers of infectious agents remain lifelong sources of the infection. For example, in typhoid fever someone may become a lifelong carrier of *Salmonella typhi* after surviving the disease. Hepatitis B and C, and HIV are other examples.

The *number of susceptible contacts* (*c*) is the sum of all single contacts between the sources of the infection and susceptible hosts. The greater the number of contacts the more likely it is that transmission will occur in the population, even if the coefficient of transmission is very low. In everyday practice it is impossible to estimate this parameter in a large population; however, in a closed population it is achievable. In hospital wards the contact between nurses and patients can be determined per day or per shift, thereby estimating the total number of possible transmissions (Austin and Anderson, 1999). The average contact can be estimated; it is quite usual in sexually transmitted diseases to estimate it by the average number of partner changes (May and Anderson, 1987).

The *frequency of the susceptible person* (*S*) in the population influences the population transmission. The proportion of immune persons in a population is called *herd immunity*, which marks the end of the transmission process. For each infection there is a threshold below which there are not enough susceptible hosts to maintain the transmission in a population. This threshold is called the *herd immunity threshold* (HIT), that is the proportion of the population that needs to be immune for an infection to become stable, i.e. each case leads to a single new case.

Several types of measures have been developed in order to estimate the population transmission:

- the basic case reproduction ratio
- the net case reproduction ratio
- the attack rate
- the secondary attack rate
- the incidence measures.

The *basic case reproduction ratio* (R_0) is the key parameter of successful transmission at the population level, which is the average number of new cases (successful transmission) originated by one infectious source in a totally susceptible population. In practice it can be measured if an infectious agent is introduced into a closed society (say an island, or hospital ward) where it has been absent for generations, or in experimental circumstances. Its value is the function of:

- the transmissibility in a single contact (β)
- the contact pattern and intensity, i.e. the number of contacts (c)
- the duration of the infectiousness (D).

Mathematically: $R_0 = \beta \times c \times D$

Thus the value of R_0 changes according to its components, especially the contact pattern, and its intensity may change in different populations. For example, for gonorrhoea $\beta = 0.35$ to transmit the *Neisseria gonorrhoeae* from a female to a male, and $D = 60$ days. If she contacts one new susceptible male every day then $R_0 = 0.35 \times 60 \times 1 = 21$ newly infected male cases can be expected. If she contacts three susceptible males per day then R_0 will be 63 new male cases.

The *net case reproduction ratio* (R) is the average number of new cases produced by one infectious source in a population composed of both immune and susceptible persons. If the population is totally susceptible then $R_0 = R$. If the infection produces immunity the transmission is constrained by the number of immune persons in a population, so R is less then R_0. That is why the net case reproduction ratio is a function of four components, of which three are common with the basic case reproduction ratio and the fourth is the proportion of susceptible persons in the population (S). If the level of contact is the same for the infectious cases between susceptible and immune individuals, then mathematically: $R_0 = R/S$.

The net case reproduction ratio is an important measure that is used for infection control programmes. If the transmission is stable, i.e. if every case leads to only one new case then $R = 1$. If R is less than one then the transmission is decreasing at the population level, because on average each case leads to less then one new case.

When the transmission is stable ($R = 1$) then the herd immunity threshold, i.e. the proportion of immune persons needed ($1 - S$) for stability, can be estimated if R_0 is known using the formula: $R_0 = 1/S$. For example, if R_0 of an infection is equal to ten then $10 = 1/S$, and $S = 0.1$, and the HIT is $1 - 0.1 = 0.9$, meaning that 90% of a population must be immune for the infection to be stable. If the infection is vaccine-preventable then the vaccination coverage should render more than 90% of the population immune to eliminate the infectious agent from the population.

Both the basic and net case reproduction ratios provide measures of the transmission between hosts in a single interval, which needs the chain of transmission to be drawn. But they do not give information about the occurrence (the absolute number of cases) of an infection, or cases relative to a baseline population where they come from – just the absolute number of new cases expected from a single contact with one case. In two identical baseline populations with stable transmission ($R = 1$) the overall occurrence can nevertheless be different. For example, 1000 existing cases with $R = 1$ produce 1000 new cases, while 100 cases with $R = 1$ give only 100 new cases, and as the baseline is identical the occurrence will be higher in the population where more cases are able to initiate the transmission of an infectious agent.

To estimate the reproduction ratios, the homologous stage of the infection (first specific clinical signs: rash, etc.) should be defined, which is characteristic only for the clinical outcomes but not for inapparent infections. A further screening is needed – if inapparent secondary cases occur – to find all secondary cases who have been in contact with a primary case in order to estimate these measures.

The *attack rate* is defined as the proportion of 'attacked' cases in a population per event. This term comes from the general meaning of the word 'attack': 'An acute episode of disease or disordered function, such as seizure, faint, or stroke' (Churchill's, 1989, p. 184). In infection control, it relates to an event (usually an outbreak situation) and not to a period of time. An outbreak of food poisoning among those who are exposed to a specific food is an example. Epidemiologically it is not a rate – it is a true proportion, estimating the probability or risk of being infected or attacked (see Chapter 7 and Elandt-Johnson, 1975). This measure is widely used in hospital settings to define the initial transmission on a ward. However, there is always a possibility of several chains of infection from multiple sources of an infectious agent.

The *secondary attack rate* is the proportion of 'attacked' cases among persons in contact with a case (usually called the primary case) within a closed community (household, hospital ward, nursery, etc.). This measure is also close to the net reproduction ratio (like the attack rate), with the difference that the number of new cases is expressed per unit of the exposed baseline population. In practice the number of contact-immune persons, and thus the number of secondary cases, is limited by the number of the exposed population, and it can therefore be much less than the maximum transmission potential of an infectious agent within an indefinitely large population. If the contact is uniform in the population then the non-attacked cases are immune persons. Multiple sources of the infection should be excluded and the homologous stage is needed for appropriate calculation, which is difficult if an infection has an inapparent outcome. This is the case for many types of HAI, especially those of bacterial origin; for example, *Klebsiella pneumoniae* may cause pneumonia, sepsis or urinary tract infection and even an inapparent outcome. In this case it is difficult to estimate the secondary attack rate or basic and net reproduction rates.

Incidence measures are discussed in Chapter 7. They estimate the overall transmission of an infectious agent by the occurrence of new cases per unit of time (week, month, year) or the average speed of an infectious agent passing through a population. The incidence measures estimate the number of all successful transmissions regardless of how many new cases occur per single infectious source.

The occurrence of an infection can be different in consecutive periods of time, reflecting any changes in successful transmission. It can be:

* sporadic
* endemic
* epidemic
* pandemic.

Sporadic cases occur occasionally, showing an irregular pattern with periods when no new cases are found. Often the chain of infection cannot be drawn up for sporadic cases because the source is not known. However, it is important to recognize that when a new infected case is found, a reservoir (source) must always exist in the environment, even if it cannot be identified during the investigation.

An *endemic level* shows persistent occurrence of the infection in each consecutive calendar period. The net reproduction ratio is equal to or very close to one, with minimal fluctuation between periods, i.e. the infection is stable. The usual activity of transmission gives the baseline level of the occurrence, which is called the expected level. In other words it is the *trend* of the occurrence of an infection. Incidence measures serve to estimate the endemic level (see Chapter 7). This level can be different for different locations due to variations in the number of the initial sources of infection. If the incidence cannot be calculated then the absolute number of cases per unit of time is acceptable; however, it is unable to estimate the risk and it can be used only in a very small population.

Different clones may circulate within a population, each contributing to the expected level. If data are available about the clonal types of individual micro-organisms then the similarities and differences of the strains can be used to discover the clone(s) responsible for maintaining the endemic level. If different clones are found then the endemy is multiclonal, and the weight of the dominant clones can be determined. If one clone circulates in a population the endemy is monoclonal.

An *epidemic* is when the occurrence of an infection becomes higher than the expected level in a defined population (Last, 1995, p. 54). Depending on the availability of the data about the expected level, three approaches can be used to define an epidemic in local situations:

- statistical approach
- threshold method (tolerance level)
- clustering approach.

The *statistical approach* requires that an increase in the occurrence above the expected level should be statistically significant in mathematical terms compared with an earlier period. For this, the risk estimated by the cumulative incidence or incidence density measures can be used (see Chapter 7). It can be used if data on the baseline occurrence are collected over quite a long period to obtain the expected level.

The *threshold method* is used when cases are not numerous enough to detect a statistically significant difference in the occurrence, but where the elevated level suggests an increased transmission. The level of tolerance can be determined locally, taking into account the previous data. Incidence measures (see Chapter 7), or the number of absolute cases per unit of time, can be used for defining the exact level of tolerance.

A *cluster of cases* is defined as those cases that are closely related by any characteristics (Last, 1995, p. 30). The term 'cluster' may be used for any kind of health-related event, but in the terminology of the transmission of infectious agents a cluster consists of those cases that are infected by the same microbial clone. It also requires an epidemiological association between cases in time and space, i.e. direct or indirect contact. The cluster approach does not require detailed baseline data – the absolute number of cases may be used for this purpose.

However, clustering may occur in both endemic and epidemic situations and the word 'clustering' is sometimes used to avoid using more alarmist terms such as 'epidemic' or 'outbreak'. Careful use of these terms is advised to avoid public confusion.

An epidemic is the result of a sudden increase of transmission at the population level due to any of the following:

- a sudden increase in the amount of an infectious agent:
  - an increase in the existing number of reservoirs of infection (poor control)
  - the introduction of an agent into a geographical area where it has not existed before
  - a shift towards longer infectiousness among infectious sources
- an enhanced mode of transmission:
  - an increase in the probability (coefficient) of transmission during contact
  - changing patterns of contact in the population – an increase in the frequency of contacts with a higher transmission coefficient in the population
  - an increase in the intensity (number) of contacts
- an increase in the number of susceptible hosts:
  - an increase in the wane of immunity at the population level
  - an increased flow (migration) of susceptible people into the population.

As mentioned above, if the number of infectious sources is constant in a population then the net reproduction ratio is elevated in an epidemic situation, exceeding one. At the National Institute of Traumatology, Budapest, three new cases of an infection (e.g. MRSA) per week in a ward is defined as the threshold of an epidemic. This is based on the net reproduction ratio because at least three cases need to be found for R to exceed one, i.e. one case generates another two new cases. One new case is hardly acceptable as an epidemic, as others have suggested (Wenzel et al., 1998). The occurrence of two associated cases does not necessarily mean an epidemic.

It is a careless expression to speak of an 'epidemic of pneumonia' or 'epidemic of a wound infection' because the infectious disease cannot be transmitted – only the infectious agent. When referring to an epidemic the exact name of the infectious agent should be specified, e.g. an epidemic of pneumonia caused by *Mycoplasma pneumoniae*, or an epidemic of wound infection caused by *Staphylococcus aureus*.

Pseudo-epidemic is the term used when an epidemic is declared but does not exist. It is a most undesirable phenomenon in infection control (Weinstein and Stamm, 1977; Morris et al., 1995). It may occur as the result of a false epidemiological association between cases for several reasons:

- specimen processing:
  - contamination during collection and transport
  - contamination in the laboratory
  - microbiological misclassification of cases:
    - the species is not correctly identified
    - poor discriminatory power of the microbiological method of typing
- the established contact between the cases is false.

Investigation of any epidemic begins with the exclusion of the possibility of pseudo-epidemic. Avoidance of pseudo-epidemic is achieved by strict quality control of specimen collection, transport, laboratory identification with highly sensitive and specific typing, and careful investigation of the cases.

A *pandemic* is defined as the epidemic occurrence of an infection in different geographic areas of the world. For HAI this term is not widely used, even if the occurrence is worldwide.

Transmission characteristics of HAI

Transmission of infectious agents in health care settings follows the same general rules as described above. However, the contact pattern may be different according to the specificity of the health care (see Figure 3.8):

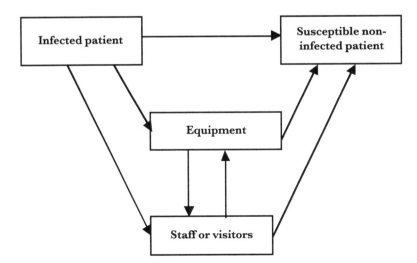

Figure 3.8. Relationship of patients, staff and visitors in the chain of infection in hospitals (arrow shows the transmission of an infectious agent).

- Direct and indirect contact between medical staff and patients daily is unavoidable due to the active nature of medical work.
- Staff may play a role in the transmission of infectious agents both as the source and as the vehicle.
- Contacts among patients may also occur directly or indirectly.
- Visitors come into contact with patients and staff.

The intensity and type of contacts may differ among wards, with different hazards of transmitting infectious agents being influenced by the following factors:

- decreased self-reliance of the patients:
    - age – paediatric, newborn wards, geriatric patients, etc.
    - consciousness and behaviour of patients – psychiatric illness
    - severity of the underlying disease
    - decreased mobility – injuries
- type and frequency of the medical procedures required.

The population of health care settings is dynamic: patients are admitted and discharged, staff and visitors enter and leave the settings. Any infectious agent can be imported into a hospital, transmitted within it or exported into the community or to another hospital. Staff within health care settings can be permanent reservoirs of such micro-organisms (Cookson et al., 1989). Intercontinental spread of infectious agents has also been documented (Oliveira et al., 1998).

Association of an infectious disease from an endogenous source and the chain of infection

An *infectious disease from an endogenous source* is where the disease develops from the autogen (endogenous) microbial flora of a host having been infected inapparently before, but not within, the maximum incubation period characteristic of the agent.

If the disease develops within the maximum incubation period after exposure to the infectious agent, then such an infectious disease is referred to as an *infectious disease from an exogenous source*.

Human individuals will have been exposed to many infectious agents since birth, and different microbes colonize the human host, thereby contributing to the body flora (see Chapter 1). The term 'colonization' is used to describe the inapparent infection if the microbes attach to and grow on those surfaces of the human body in direct contact with the environment (skin, outer ear, mucosa of respiratory, genito-urinary and alimentary tracts) (Last, 1995, p. 85).

Human flora encompasses both apathogen and facultative pathogen micro-organisms of both bacterial and fungal origin (see Chapter 1 and Table 1.9). For example, 20% of the human population harbour *Staphylococcus aureus* on their skin, in nasal mucosa, and it can even be detected in faeces, without any sign of infection. However, *Staphylococcus aureus* is one of the most common agents of HAI originating from the endogen flora of individuals, especially in surgical wound infections (Howard et al., 1964).

Viruses – being intracellular pathogens – are not counted as part of this flora, even though they can also infect humans inapparently. Other microbes – such as prions, rickettsiae, mycoplasmae, Chlamydiae, protozoa and helminths are also not counted as part of human body flora. Thus they hardly cause primary endogenous clinical infection.

However, the build-up and exchange of flora of the human body also results from the transmission of infectious agents from external sources, coming from the environment. Furthermore, the time and place of this cannot be determined exactly in each case because originally the infection is inapparent. Studies using culture techniques have produced evidence that the flora of hospitalized patients can be replaced by so-called nosocomial microbes occurring at higher frequency in health care settings, and such flora may be responsible for late clinical infections in hospitals (Johanson et al., 1969). Patients discharged from hospital may harbour hospital pathogens indefinitely – for weeks, months or even years – until their florae have been replaced by those micro-organisms that circulate in their normal environment.

The emergence of disease from the endogenous flora occurs as a result of several factors (see Figure 2.1):

- the natural increase of invasiveness (virulence) of the micro-organisms in the flora
- an artificial break in the protective barriers during invasive procedures at those sites where the flora occurs (skin, mucosa of the sites having an external lumen to the environment)
- decrease of local defence mechanisms.'

The importance of this type of infection lies in the development of a disease, and it is quite common within the community (because of injuries) and it accounts for a large number infections in hospitals as a result of invasive medical procedures.

Summary

This chapter has set out the essentials of the transmission concept of infectious disease at the individual and population levels. The following points should be highlighted:

- The concept of the transmission of infectious agents is fundamental and is used equally in infectious diseases in both the community and in hospitals.
- Transmission can be characterized qualitatively by the type (mode) of transmission. An official report of the American Public Health Association, Control of Communicable Diseases Manual contains detailed information about the mode of transmission of infectious agents of human interest (Chin., 2000). This book is the standard-bearer for infection control practitioners, but can also be useful for clinicians.
- The spread of infectious agents can also be characterized quantitatively by using reproduction measures and different mathematical models. This needs some mathematical knowledge, which seems to be far from clinical practice, but it is advisable to understand the basic principles of the dynamics of infections because it is the basis of infection control, and clinicians in hospital are part of such control measures. Actively changing the contact pattern toward a lower coefficient of transmission (e.g. wearing gloves during patient care) or decreasing the proportion of susceptible persons (e.g. by immunization) or reducing the contact to a minimum, are based on reproduction theory in order to decrease transmission and the number of new cases. The effect of such measures has been demonstrated in practice (see Chapters 5 and 6).

CHAPTER 4

Definitions and general characteristics of infections in hospitals

Aims of definitions in medicine

The first and essential part of both preventive and therapeutic medicine is the clear distinction of one case from another. 'Case – a person in the population or study group identified as having the particular disease, health disorder, or condition under investigation' (Last, 1995, p. 22).

Case definition is a set of standard criteria (clinical signs and complementary diagnostic characteristics) to distinguish one health-related event from another, regardless of infectious or non-infectious origin. The purpose of the standardization of the criteria is to ensure that each case is diagnosed in the same way – even if the diagnosis is made by a different person, at a different time and location – in order to make the cases comparable.

Case definitions are important in two respects:

- clinical – for clinicians to make the correct diagnosis of the health-related event, choosing the appropriate type of therapy, if needed
- preventive (epidemiological) – for preventive measures specific to the health-related event.

Diagnostic procedures use an algorithm to define a case; this is called *differential diagnosis*. It is defined as 'The process of making a diagnosis by comparing and analyzing the similarities and differences between the signs, symptoms, and other findings associated particularly with two or more diseases sharing the certain characteristics' (Churchill's, 1989, p. 510). The sum of all the clinical signs (symptoms) is called a *syndrome*. Differential diagnosis is based on syndromes and laboratory diagnostic procedures. One health event is clearly distinguishable from another if it has specific distinguishing features (a syndrome or symptoms). Where symptoms and laboratory findings are common to two or more health events, these are called general findings. Sometimes it is difficult to make a correct diagnosis in a case because there are similar clinical signs for the different diseases, or there is a lack of sufficiently sensitive and specific diagnostic procedures (see Chapter 1). This results in a categorization of cases according to the degree of certainty of the correctness of the diagnosis:

- confirmed case
- probable case
- suspect case.

A *confirmed case* is when we are sure that a person has a specific health-related event. In the case of infections it is essential to identify the infectious agent, which is usually confirmed by microbiological investigation. Some infections can be confirmed based only on clinical findings, with no need for microbiological confirmation, for example erysipelas caused by *Streptococcus pyogenes*. But for inapparent cases microbiological confirmation will be necessary.

A *probable case* is when the case is not confirmed, owing to incompleteness of the available essential criteria for a differential diagnosis, and there can therefore be only an assumption about the exact type of health-related event. For infections, lack of essential microbiological confirmation will require the case to be designated as probable, and the diagnosis will be based only on the non-specific clinical signs (a syndrome). This category is not applicable to an inapparent infection unless there is strong evidence that the case was in contact with a confirmed case with a high probability of transmission, or if the case seems likely to be the source of the infectious agent. A clinically compatible case is a probable case when the clinical syndrome is generally compatible with the disease.

A *suspect case* is similar to a probable case, with the distinction that there are even fewer criteria than are needed to define a probable case. For example, measles may be suspected from a rash and fever (Wharton et al., 1990).

For clinicians, it is desirable to achieve confirmation of diagnosis because the quality of therapy depends on this. However, for the purposes of experts in public health or infection control, the case definitions of both confirmed and probable cases may be acceptable, according to the main public health purposes of a given situation:

- A 'sensitive' or 'loose' case definition is used if it is important to find *every possible* case (including probable and suspect cases), not missing anyone, together with confirmed cases.
- A 'specific' or 'strict' definition is used to identify only confirmed cases of the particular infection.

However, for medico-legal purposes a 'strict' definition is required in an individual case because uncertainty should be avoided, which is inherent in the categories of probable and suspect cases.

Requirements for the definition of hospital-acquired infections

The definition of any infection acquired during health care is important for public health and for medico-legal purposes, in order to distinguish them from infections originating outside the hospital. Furthermore, clear and uniform definitions are required to enable comparable estimates of the magnitude of hospital-acquired infection both within and among hospitals (see Chapter 7). Inconsistency of definitions used in different periods may lead to inaccurate comparisons being made. Measures of hospital-acquired infection reflect the individual risk of developing an infection during health care. Two requirements are essential to determine the presence of HAI:

- whether the patient has an infection at all (case definitions of infection)
- whether the infection is associated with (or a consequence of) the health care.

Case definitions for hospital-acquired infection are the same as those for clinical or public health purposes, the only difference being their hospital dependence. Two types of infection occur in hospitals, depending on their origin:

- imported infection or community-acquired infection (CAI)
- hospital-acquired infection (HAI) or nosocomial infection.

Types of definition of hospital-acquired infection

Many different definitions of HAI can be found in the scientific literature to distinguish such infection from CAI, which reflects the complexity and difficulties of defining these infections precisely (Garner et al., 1988; Dorland's, 1988, p. 1052; Horan et al., 1992a, 1992b; Glenister et al., 1992b; Last, 1995, p. 115). Indeed, the issue seems so important that duplicate publishing has even been observed from the same authors (Horan et al., 1992a, 1992b). Crowe and Cooke tried to compare the existing definitions by emphasizing the differences between them, so confirming the lack of a uniform definition system (Crowe and Cooke, 1998).

Definitions of HAI fall into two broad systems:

• general definitions
• specific definitions.

General definitions of hospital-acquired infection

General definitions describe HAI according to common features, i.e. any infection originating in health care. They are very simple and straightforward and are widely used. General definitions of HAI are based on the infectious process of clinical infection, and two types have been described:

• incubation period based
• 'cut-off' point based.

Incubation period based definition requires knowledge of the incubation period of each type of infection. Hospital acquired infection: 'An infection originating in a medical facility, e.g. occurring in a patient in a hospital or other health care facility in whom the infection was not present or incubating at the time of admission' (Last, 1995, p. 115). Despite being a most frequently quoted definition, it should be applied very carefully:

• If the term 'infection' is applied only to clinical infections then it is disease oriented and ignores inapparent infections; this should be made clear (Last, 1995, p. 115).
• There is no precisely defined range of incubation and latent periods for many infections (for example, MRSA) and the beginning of clinical infection may not enable the exact time of the exposure to be determined, and whether it happened before or after admission.
• It does not explain the hospital origin of a clinical infection that develops due to the consequences of medical procedures in a patient initially colonized with an infectious agent at the time of admission.

- Superinfection by another infectious agent at the site of infection, which can happen in hospitals, is ignored.

The synonym for 'hospital-acquired infection' is the term 'nosocomial infection' (Last, 1995, p. 115). The word 'nosocomial' is of Greek origin: *noso(s)* = sickness + *komeein* = to attend, pertaining or acquired in a hospital (Churchill's, 1989, p. 1287).

Cut-off point based definition is the other widely accepted definition of HAI, which adds a time limit ('cut-off point') to the general definition: hospital-acquired infection is so called if it develops after admission to hospital, and the patient was not in the incubation period on admission, or if it develops 48 hours or more after admission (Dorland's, 1988, p. 1152; Coello et al., 1997). This definition compensates for the disadvantages of the general definition, adding the cut-off point for those infections where the exact value of incubation period cannot be determined. This two-day interval is arbitrary and sometimes it is prolonged up to 72 hours. The following additional considerations are recommended, using this limit in order to avoid confusion and taking into account the above comment:

- It is not necessarily the case that a patient will acquire an infectious agent two or three days after admission, even if the likelihood of this is increasing.
- Inapparent infection originating in hospital should be regarded as HAI.

Definitions of HAIs relying only on the incubation period have limitations:

- In correct use, the term 'infection' covers both inapparent and symptomatic infections (Last, 1995, p. 85). This distinction should be maintained. Procedures without which the clinical infection would not develop are an *essential* part of the development of HAI, even if the patient was already colonized at the time of admission, i.e. was infected with the infectious agent causing the disease before admission. In this case, the infection was acquired outside the hospital, but the clinical development is hospital-dependent. The best example is the postoperative surgical wound infection, where the development of the clinical infection is caused by the endogenous bacterial flora (*Staphylococcus* or other species) of the operated patient.
- Furthermore, it is essential to include both the inapparent and the clinical cases in a system of definition for public health purposes because in

routine infection control *all* new cases should be included for the estimation of the transmission of an infectious agent (see Chapter 7). If only clinical cases are counted then such definitions may lead to an underestimation of transmission, by ignoring the fact that new inapparent cases are also the result of transmission. Colonized and clinical cases are of equal importance in infection control, both being sources of an infectious agent. The magnitude of this underestimation is related to the ratio of the clinical cases to the unrecognized (silent) inapparent cases. If specimens are not taken for microbiological diagnosis at the time of admission it is difficult later to define the time and place of acquisition of the 'silent' infectious agent, which may lead to the misclassification of imported cases as nosocomial ones. Such misclassification can also happen if the patient is initially infected at admission but the microbiological result is falsely negative.

There are guidelines that recommend screening patients on admission if there is a possibility that they can import an infectious agent into the health care setting from outside where the agent is endemic, which also suggests that modified definitions are necessary for such situations. For example, in the case of methicillin-resistant *Staphylococcus aureus* (MRSA) it is important to distinguish imported cases from locally acquired cases (Hospital Infection Society and British Society, 1990; Glupczinsky et al., 1994; Working Party, 1998). This can be seen in Figure 4.1, where the patterns of infection caused by MRSA at the National Institute of Traumatology, Budapest, are illustrated.

Cluster analysis with geno- and phenotyping of cultured strains might be a helpful complementary method in the nosocomial classification of infections, especially if specimens are not taken at the time of admission but later, and show true positive results (Maslow et al., 1993). However, this is not done in everyday practice for several reasons:

- Cultured strains from different cases should be stored to distinguish different clones.
- Strains should be classifiable using standard typing methods.
- Typing should have very high discriminatory power.
- It needs more expensive laboratory support, which increases the cost.

Disease-free patients admitted primarily from the community are usually not screened for cost/benefit reasons. However, if a patient is transferred

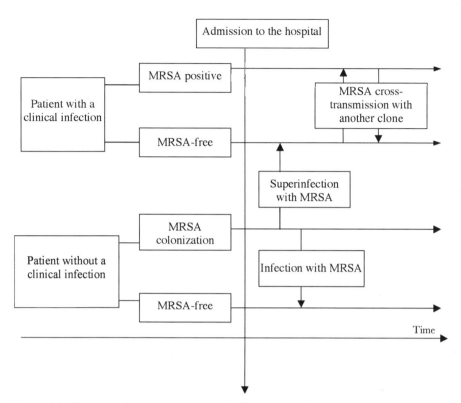

Figure 4.1. The transmission patterns of methicillin-resistant Staphylococcus aureus (MRSA) among patients observed at the National Institute of Traumatology, Budapest, Hungary.

from one hospital to another it is advisable to screen for the most frequent nosocomial microbes. Additionally, screening of high-risk groups has been found to be effective because it is more likely that they harbour microbes that are important in hospital infection control.

The transmission of infectious agents with different outcomes and the presence of medical procedures may result in a combination of different patterns of nosocomial infection, which needs to be taken into account when formulating definitions. Two main patterns of nosocomial infection can be distinguished:

- the patient acquires an infection via the transmission of an infectious agent in a hospital
- the patient imports the infectious agent inapparently into the hospital, but a clinical infection subsequently develops as a result of medical intervention.

If the aim is to give a general definition of nosocomial infections and to describe their nature, both transmission and procedures are essential elements of such infections and must be considered together. This is attempted in the following definition:

> An infection is defined as nosocomial if an infectious agent is acquired from a source of the healthcare setting external to the patient regardless of the outcome of the infection, or where a medical procedure is essential for the development of a clinical infection from an endogenous source, regardless of the place of acquisition of the infectious agent.

In accordance with the concept of transmission, imported infections can be defined as follows:

> An imported infection is an infection that is present at the time of admission, regardless of the presence of any clinical signs, or when the clinical signs develop in a shorter time than the maximum incubation period from the time of admission.

Specific definitions of hospital-acquired infection

Several attempts have been made since the 1960s to provide uniform specific definitions for each HAI by the Centers for Disease Control and Prevention, Atlanta (CDC) in order to make the collection of data comparable across different projects (Garner, et al., 1988; Haley et al., 1980b):

- Comprehensive Hospital Infections Project (CHIP) from 1969 to 1972;
- National Nosocomial Infections Study (NNIS) from 1970 until 1974;
- Study of the Efficacy of Nosocomial Infection Control (SENIC) in 1975-1976.

The CDC in 1988 published a new set of definitions for the most common nosocomial infections, based on modifications of earlier definitions (Garner et al., 1988). This definition system can be characterized as follows:

- it defines the main nosocomial infections according to the anatomical site of the infection and the clinical features
- the term 'infection' is taken to be equivalent to 'infectious disease' and is not coherent with the definition of the term 'infection' given by Last and colleagues (Last, 1995, p. 85), and the term 'colonization' is used for inapparent infections

- it also recognizes an infection as nosocomial if the aetiology of the existing infection at the same anatomical site changes, and the new pathogen cultured from this site is recognized as a further cause of the disease
- inapparent infections originating in hospital are omitted from the definition.

Despite the vulnerable points of the existing systems of definition, their role cannot be ignored in hospitals because they are currently the most affordable way to keep infection control systematic and consistent. However, it is essential to declare what kinds of definitions are used in the collected data in order to make valid comparisons with both retrospective and prospective data (see Chapter 7).

Classification of hospital acquired infection

Nosocomial infections are strongly associated with health care settings that are designed for carrying out medical procedures. Any medical intervention, whether it is done in a health care setting or outside, harbours a potential hazard for the development of complications in the patient, which can be non-infectious or infectious.

The patterns of nosocomial infections are the same as for infections outside hospital (i.e. influenza, dysentery, etc.), and even the mechanism of wound infections is the same. The difference lies in the frequency of the invasive procedures between health care settings and the community. In hospitals – especially in developed countries – the relative frequency of procedure-dependent HAI among all infections is higher than in the community.

Medical procedures can be classified into two main categories:

- diagnostic procedures
- therapeutic procedures.

The common feature of both types is that they involve active physical contact between the staff and the patient. This promotes the transmission of infectious agents.

Diagnostic procedures are carried out to diagnose the underlying and concomitant disease(s) of the patient. They are of three broad types:

- physical examination
- laboratory investigation
- imaging techniques.

Therapeutic procedures aim to restore the normal physiological state by prescribing drugs, by operating on the patient, or by other methods.

Both diagnostic and therapeutic procedures can be further divided into:

- non-invasive procedures
- invasive procedures.

Non-invasive procedures (single X-ray, ultrasonography, oral tablets, etc.) do not lead to injury of the barriers (skin and mucosa), and their mechanical resistance against infectious agents will not be altered. However, the function of the immune system may be compromised by such non-invasive procedures as steroids, immune-suppression, X-ray therapy, etc., which may cause an increased susceptibility to infections among such patients.

Invasive procedures lead to a break in the barriers, both dermal and mucosal, which opens the gates for the infectious agents to enter the deep tissues of the body, even for those agents that have low affinity for invasiveness (see Chapter 2). In medicine such procedures are done consciously and unavoidably (injections, surgical operations, endoscopy, diagnostic punctures, etc.) for the benefit of patients. By the beginning of the twenty-first century medicine has become more invasive and more aggressive, increasing the proportion of invasive procedures and thus increasing the risk of complications.

Outside health care, injuries to barriers occur naturally during accidental traumas or through conscious behaviour (crime, attempted suicide, intravenous drug use, social and cultural behaviour, tattoos). The pattern of such infections will be the same as for HAI because of the invasive proced-ures involved. Patients admitted to hospital with dirty open wounds due to trauma will develop infections more frequently than those exposed to aseptic conditions in hospital (Howard et al., 1964; Cruse and Foord, 1980).

For the purposes of practical infection control, infections in hospitals can be classified in several ways according to the possible influence of susceptibility, and depending on the procedures employed. This is important for the decision-making processes in the prevention of HAI (see Figure 4.2).

Invasive procedures are uniform in health care settings throughout the world, which explains why the occurrence and pattern of procedure-dependent HAI is similar; furthermore, the natural flow of infections shows many similarities. This results in the fact that the same ten HAI are the

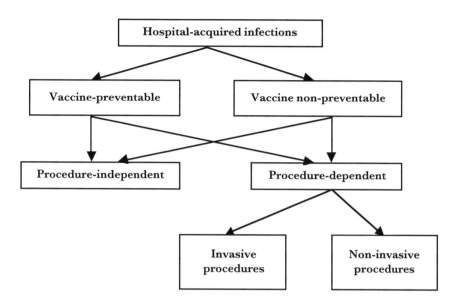

Figure 4.2. Classification of nosocomial infections.

most common in every hospital, and among them the following are the most important (see Chapter 6):

- urinary tract infections
- wound infections
- pneumonia
- alimentary tract infections
- bloodstream infections.

Risk factors and the preventability of hospital-acquired infection

Hospitals in different countries, and even different wards within a hospital, may differ in the magnitude of invasive procedures employed, which explains the difference of the occurrence of HAI associated with medical procedures. The higher the frequency of invasive procedures among admitted patients the greater the magnitude of the complications. This explains the higher occurrence of HAI in intensive care units (ICU), and in surgical services (abdominal, chest, urogenital, trauma, neurosurgery, etc.).

The expected level and preventability of HAI is influenced by many factors that can be grouped according to the:

- prevalence of susceptible patients admitted to the hospital, susceptible staff and susceptible visitors
- probability of being exposed to an infectious agent in hospital, i.e. the occurrence of the infectious agent
- nature of the infection:
  - transmission patterns and characteristics
  - clinical patterns of the infection
- prevalence of medical procedures – both invasive and non-invasive
- frequency of endogenous or exogenous risk factors predisposing to HAI.

'*Susceptibility*' in population science means that everybody in the population has a certain chance of being infected. However, susceptibility can be limited when only a part of the population is susceptible to an infection for some reason, for example those who are unvaccinated. It is possible to characterize any population according to its susceptibility to infection.

The *probability of exposure* to an infectious agent depends on the distribution of different microbes in the hospital microbial flora – called 'nosocomial flora' – where the patient is admitted, and depends also on the imported micro-organisms. This influences the aetiological distribution of HAI, which is called 'microbial trends'.

The *nature of the infection* (transmission features, procedure-dependence, or both) determines the mechanism of the development of an infection, and the clinical patterns (see Chapters 2 and 3).

The *prevalence of medical procedures* influences the occurrence of procedure-associated HAI directly. In hospitals, injections, intravenous catheters, urinary tract catheters, surgical operations and mechanical ventilation are the most frequently used invasive procedures. The higher the prevalence of invasive procedures, the higher the expected frequency.

Invasive procedures induce a circle called a 'circulus vitiosus' where a disorder of vital organs needs invasive procedures that are risk factors promoting the development of infection. Infections, especially pneumonia or sepsis, will lead to further decrease of the function of vital organs, which needs further invasive procedures, or the maintenance of earlier ones (see Figure 4.3). It is extremely difficult to interrupt this circle, which requires prompt antibiotic and other treatment. Thus successful clinical management of an infection may prevent further HAI by interrupting the circle.

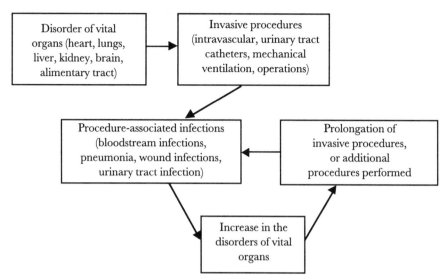

Figure 4.3. Role of invasive procedures in maintaining hospital-acquired infections.

The *frequency of endogenous and exogenous risk factors* also influences the occurrence of HAI. Risk factors have been described generally in Chapter 1 as determinants of HAI. They have been extensively researched. Both the endogenous and exogenous risk factors can be *specific*, which is characteristic of a particular infection, and can be *general*, which contributes to a higher risk of all types of infections. The following general endogenous risk factors have been studied in HAI:

- age
- severity of the underlying disease
- length of hospitalization
- drugs.

Age has been found to be a risk factor (Celis et al., 1988; Saviteer et al., 1988; Tess et al., 1993). A quadratic function was found between age and HAI in a simple mathematical model, where the occurrence of HAI was higher in both very young and elderly people (Goonatilake, 1985). The same quadratic relationship was found between age and nasal carriage of *Staphylococcus aureus* (Ayliffe et al., 1977).

Severity of underlying diseases is the second most studied risk factor. Different systems have been proposed in order to predict the effect of underlying diseases on HAI:

- ASA Physical Status Classification

- fatality of underlying disease
- Glasgow coma scale
- APACHE II score system.

The *ASA (American Society of Anaesthesiologist) Physical Status Classification* was first introduced by a committee of the American Society of Anaesthetists composed of doctors E.A. Rovenstine, M. Saklad and I.B. Taylor in 1941 in order to predict the outcome of surgical interventions (Saklad, 1941). Originally six classes were defined, and later modifications were made by several well-known scientists (and anonymously) (Dripps et al., 1961; Keats, 1978; Owens et al., 1978). The final version has been widely used since 1974 after rhetorical changes, which consists of five classes (Owens et al., 1978; Table 4.1). Despite the wide use of the ASA system, it has some disadvantages:

- The classification is subjective because no objectively verifiable physiological parameters have been determined, which leads to low repeatability.
- The most frequent misclassification occurs by classifying Class 2 patients as Class 3, and vice versa, owing to subjective decisions about the 'incapacitating systemic disease'.

Table 4.1. The ASA (American Society of Anesthesiologists) physical status classification

Class 1	A normally healthy patient
Class 2	A patient with mild systemic disease
Class 3	A patient with severe systemic disease that is not incapacitating
Class 4	A patient with an incapacitating systemic disease that is a constant threat to life
Class 5	A moribund patient who is not expected to survive for 24 hours with or without operation

Source: after Owens et al., 1978.

Severity of underlying disease was the second system used to estimate the risk of HAI by grading the severity of the underlying disease according to the fatality outcome:

- non-fatal
- ultimately fatal
- rapidly fatal.

This system has mainly been applied not for risk assessment of HAI but for quality assurance programmes, replacing the term 'severity of illness' by 'case-mix index' (Jencks and Dobson, 1987). The main use of this index is to estimate the hospital costs, which, of course, may increase with the greater severity of underlying diseases.

The *Glasgow coma scale (GCS)* was introduced by Teasdale and Jennett to evaluate the function of the central nervous system, and it is widely used in neurosurgery for patients with neurological damage from any cause (Teasdale and Jennett, 1974; Teasdale et al., 1979). The essence of the GCS is a scoring method of investigating the response function of the central nervous system (CNS) using eye, verbal and motor responses (see Table 4.2).

Table 4.2. Glasgow Coma Score (GCS)

Neurological responses and corresponding scores					
Eye opening (E)		**Best verbal response (V)**		**Best motor response (M)**	
spontaneous	4	orientated	5	obey commands	6
to sound	3	confused	4	localize	5
to pain	2	inappropriate	3	flexion: normal	4
never	1	incomprehensible	2	flexion: abnormal	3
		none	1	extension	2
				nil	1

Source: after Teasdale and Jennett, 1974; Teasdale et al., 1979.

The GCS reflects the severity of the injury to the CNS and thus indirectly estimates the necessary degree of invasive procedures on the CNS and other organs of vital importance (e.g. liquor drainage, mechanical ventilation, etc.). The highest possible score is 15, which indicates a much better quality of survival than remaining vegetative. The lower the GCS the higher the risk of further hospitalization, and thus of acquiring HAI because the likelihood of survival in a vegetative state is high. It is one of the most widely used score systems in intensive care units (ICU).

Acute Physiology and Chronic Health Evaluation II (APACHE II) is the most extensively used system in ICUs despite its complexity and time-consuming method of calculation. Basically, the APACHE II score is the result of the sum of two sub-score systems (Rowan et al., 1993a, 1993b):

• acute physiology score
• age and history of chronic conditions.

The *acute physiology score (APS)* requires knowledge of rectal temperature, mean blood pressure, heart rate, respiratory rate, oxygenization, arterial pH, serum sodium, serum potassium, serum creatinine, haematocrit, white bloodcell count, and the Glasgow coma scale (see Table 4.3).

Table 4.3. Points in acute physiology score (APS)

Physiological parameter	Scores								
	4	3	2	1	0	1	2	3	4
Rectal temperature (°C)	≥41.0	39.0–40.9		38.5–38.9	36.0–38.4	34.0–35.9	32.0–33.9	30.0–31.9	≤29.9
Mean blood pressure (mmHg)	≥160	130–159	110–129		70–109		50–69		≤49
Heart rate (ventricular response/min)	≥180	140–179	110–139		70–109		55–69	40–54	≤39
Respiratory rate (breaths/min)	≥50	35–49		25–34	12–24	10–11	6–9		≤5
Oxygenation									
I (≥50%)	≥500	350–499	200–349		<200				
II (<50%)					>70	61–70		55–60	<55
Arterial pH	≥7.70	7.60–7.69		7.50–7.59	7.33–7.49		7.25–7.32	7.15–7.24	<7.15
Serum sodium (mmol/l)	≥180	160–179	155–159	150–154	130–149		120–129	111–119	≤110
Serum potassium (mmol/l)	≥7.0	6.0–6.9		5.5–5.9	3.5–5.4	3.0–3.4	2.5–2.9		<2.5
Serum creatinine (mg/100ml)	≥3.5	2.0–3.4	1.5–1.9		0.6–1.4		<0.6		
Haematocrit	≥60		50–59.9	46–49.9	30–45.9		20–29.9		<20
White blood cell count (×10³/ml³)	≥40		20–39.9	15–19.9	3–14.9		1–2.9		<1
GCS					13–15 l				

Source: after Rowan et al., 1993a,b; GCS = Glasgow coma score.

However, the APS cannot be applied outside the ICU, thus it is not appropriate to use to estimate the risk of HAI in other departments.

Age and history of chronic conditions is a simple score system, added to APS to obtain APACHE II, which gives a higher score – i.e. higher risk – if the patient is older and if a chronic condition is present (see Table 4.4).

Table 4.4. Points assigned to age and chronic disease as part of APECHE II score

Characteristics	Score	
Age	< 45	0
	45–54	2
	55–64	3
	65–74	5
	≥ 75	6
History of chronic conditions	none	0
	elective surgical patient	2
	emergency surgical or non-surgical patient	5

Source: after Rowan et al., 1993a,b.

There is an inconsistency in the APACHE II score system because in the GCS system the higher the score the better the chances of survival, while in the APS score the higher scores on the physiological parameters (without GCS) indicate a higher risk of HAI. Adding the sub-scores – i.e. scores of the physiological parameters to the GCS – may cause confusion in the final score (see Tables 4.2, 4.3 and 4.4).

Length of hospitalization has also been studied as a risk factor for HAI. It has been found that the greater the length of hospitalization, the greater the risk of HAI (Saviteer et al., 1988; Tess et al., 1993). However, length of hospitalization can influence the risk of HAI only indirectly. Patients stay for longer periods in hospital as a result of invasive procedures necessary to treat the disorders of vital organs, which may lead to the acquisition of infections (see Figure 4.3). The expected length of stay in hospital depends on the severity of the underlying disease.

Drugs (antibiotics and immunosuppressants) can also influence the risk of HAI. Adequate antibiotic prophylaxis reduces the risk of wound infections, while its lack will result in an elevated risk (Kaiser, 1986). It is not disputable that immunosuppressants (steroids, antimyelopoetic drugs, etc.) decrease the function of the immune system of patients who are suffering from autoimmune disorders, undergoing transplantation, or being treated for neoplasm.

Exogenous general risk factors – as we saw in Chapter 1 – are those that depend on structural conditions for the prevention of HAI. The availability of those elements depends on the socioeconomic status of the particular country and area where the hospital is, and on the rational use of those resources by the hospital management.

Specific risk factors for HAI can be grouped into two main types:

- site-specific
- micro-organism-specific.

Site-specific risk factors are those that influence the risk of a specified HAI. Specific risk factors for urinary tract infections, wound infections, pneumonia, infection of the alimentary tract and bloodstream are discussed in Chapter 6.

Micro-organism-specific risk factors are those that explain the differences in the occurrence and severity of HAI caused by different species and subtypes. The role of microbiology, especially molecular biology, has been increasing in this area of research. Discovering microbes with 'unusual' resistance, increased possibility of transmission, and lethality gives a much greater insight into understanding infections in hospitals.

The prevention of HAI is a most difficult task. The difficulties are inherent in the presence of both exogenous and endogenous risk factors. The eradication of HAI is a nightmare, but the reduction of the occurrence of HAI to an optimal level can be achieved. However, clinical staff and infection control specialists should do their best to *prevent* HAI as far as possible.

Summary

This chapter has summarized the general respects of HAI, and the following points are highlighted:

- Historically, different definitions have been developed for HAI, which have advantages and disadvantages. However, in everyday practice for clinicians, the differential diagnosis of infections is the most important.
- Nosocomial infections must be accepted as a fact of life, but that is no reason not to attempt to prevent them, nor to try to mitigate their effects, and conscious action by clinicians is required.
- The more invasive the medicine, the higher the expected occurrence of HAIs.

- Controllable risk factors are a promising weapon in prevention strategy, which may vary between countries and even among hospitals, depending on the socioeconomic resources and willingness of staff to search for and eliminate such risk factors.
- Score systems (ASA, severity of underlying disease, GCS, and APACHE II and even APACHE III) have been developed to estimate the susceptibility of patients, stratifying them according to the risk scores. These score systems are used mainly for epidemiological purposes and provide some standardization for comparison of the occurrence of HAIs between hospitals, at both national and international levels. However, they hardly serve as sources of everyday practical help unless to forecast the risk of HAI at the individual level. The limitation of such score systems is that they estimate susceptibility only indirectly.

CHAPTER 5

Preventive strategies for hospital-acquired infection

Prevention of the transmission of infectious agents (isolation policy)

Isolation of infection

Isolation of infection is defined as the use of all measures that prevent the direct and indirect transmission of an infectious agent from the source or the reservoir to a recipient host. The word 'isolation' is of French-Italian origin: *isolé, isolato* = separated, apart.

Some authors use the term 'isolation' only for the separation of infected persons: 'Isolation – the separation for the period of communicability of infected persons from other persons, in such places and under such conditions as will prevent the direct or indirect conveyance of the infectious agent from infected persons to persons who are susceptible or who may spread the agent to others. This applies also to animals' (Top, 1967, p. 64).

The term 'isolation of infection' has a broader sense than the isolation of the source of the infectious agent alone, because the intervention may occur not only at the source of the infectious agent.

The term 'isolation of infectious agent' can be ambiguous as it may mean the detection of an infectious agent by a microbiological method or it may mean the separation (localization) of the agent in the environment with a preventive purpose. Thus the term 'isolation of infection' will be used in this book to avoid misunderstanding.

Isolation of infection may be achieved by the interruption of the chain of infection at any of three stages (Figure 5.1):

- isolation of the source (reservoir) of infection – separation of the infectious source so as to prevent the spread of the infectious agent to the

vehicle of transmission, or direct to the recipient host, or by decontamination of the source of infection
- interruption of the chain of infection at the mode of transmission by
decontamination of the vehicle of infection
- increasing the resistance of the recipient host against the infectious agent,
or separating it from the source or the vehicle of the infectious agent.

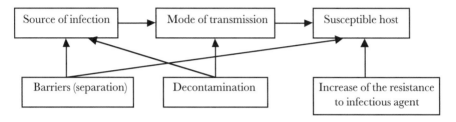

Figure 5.1. Interruption of the transmission of infectious agents.

There are two main functions of isolation, according to the relative hazard
of the transmission of the infectious agent:

- protective isolation
- infective isolation.

Protective isolation is used for immuno-compromised patients in order to protect
them from the transmission of an infectious agent from an immuno-compe-
tent person or other source to prevent the serious consequences of acquiring
an infection. This type of isolation is used, for example, in bone marrow or
kidney transplantation, when immuno-suppression is used to decrease the
function of the immune system in recipients to avoid organ rejection. It is also
used for newborn babies with congenital immune disorders.

   Infective isolation is used when the host, regardless of the immune status,
harbours a hazardous agent that is likely to transmit an infectious agent
into the environment. Here the aim is to prevent the transmission to other
possible hosts in the environment.

Isolation policy

High-quality infection control requires systematic care in the prevention of
the transmission of infectious agents among patients, health care workers
and visitors. *Isolation policy* is the term used to describe the documentation

and regulation of all measures to prevent the transmission of infectious agents. It can be regulated by law or by standards set by the national occupational safety administrative systems, with further optional regulations adopted by the local hospital infection control system.

An isolation policy must be effective. This means that the transmission path of the specific infectious agent is interrupted for both patients and staff immediately after the detection of a single case within the hospital. *Under-isolation* happens if the specific infectious agent is transmitted despite the use of precautions because of objective (inadequate precautions) or subjective (ignorance) reasons, or both. *Over-isolation* occurs if unnecessary precautions are taken for the specific agent. It is important to remember that anyone (patient, staff and visitors) may be infected inapparently and be a potential source of infectious agents, and in practice it is impossible to establish a general system of precautions to prevent transmission by every possible route. The choice of isolation precautions depends on:

- professional aspects:
  - routes of transmission of the known or suspected infectious agent
  - the relative hazard of the infection, i.e. the severity of the consequences of the infection
- economic aspects:
  - the availability of resources for health care in the specific country
  - the cost-effectiveness of precautions.

Ignacz Semmelweis was the first in medical history to mention isolation: 'It is also necessary that every maternity hospital contain several isolation rooms in order that individuals who exude decaying matter can be isolated' (Semmelweis, 1861, p. 165).

Until the 1960s special infectious disease hospitals were built worldwide to provide separate facilities for infected patients with community-acquired infections (poliomyelitis, measles, hepatitis A, etc.) who needed hospitalization owing to the severity of their illness. However, isolation was not a recommended practice in other types of hospital for patients with HAI. In the 1960s changes took place whereby simple and effective isolation techniques were recommended to be applied in all health care settings (CDC, 1970). Subsequent modifications have been made for several reasons: changes in the patient population; the appearance of HIV; recognition of the occupational aspects of infections in hospitals; changes in technology, e.g. the availability of disposable gloves, masks for use in isolation; the need for documented infection control and quality control in hospitals (Lynch et al., 1987; CDC, 1987, 1988; Lynch et al., 1990). These modifications have led to the development of four systems of isolation:

- category-specific
- disease-specific
- body substance isolation
- universal precautions.

Category-specific isolation (CSI) corresponds to the localization of the portal of exit of an infectious agent from the reservoir or source of infection. Seven categories of isolation are identified (CDC, 1970; Garner, 1996a, 1996b): strict, airborne/respiratory, protective, enteric/secretion, wound and skin, discharge, and blood. The essence of this categorization is that many infections share the same or similar transmission route. Its advantage is that it is simple, with colour-coded signs used to indicate all requirements. Many infections have more than one method of transmission and these overlap the different categories within this system. Over-isolation can occur if unnecessary precautions are taken. Revision took place in 1975 (CDC, 1975).

Disease-specific isolation (DSI) was the first major modification of CSI, made to overcome the disadvantages of having in place many different requirements for each type of infection. It takes into account the methods of transmission that are common to different infections. Despite its advantages, DSI was recommended only as an alternative system (not replacing the CSI system completely) and hospitals were allowed to develop their own systems (CDC, 1981; Garner and Simmons, 1983; Garner, 1996a).

Body substance isolation (BSI) was developed in order to decrease the transmission of nosocomial infectious agents to patients, and to reduce the transmission of agents from the patients to health care workers (Lynch et al., 1987; Lynch et al., 1990). Its essence is the use of fresh rubber gloves for each patient during contact with mucosa and non-intact skin, and wearing gloves when in contact with any moist body substances. Other barriers are used to protect the skin and clothes of health care personnel. The recommendation was that these precautions should be used for *all* patients regardless of any diagnosed or suspected infections.

Universal precautions (UP) or Universal Blood and Body Fluid Precautions were developed by combining the category-specific and body-substance isolation systems (CDC, 1988). In this recommendation the 'blood and body fluid precautions' were specified for use with *all* patients, and all body fluids were regarded as potential sources of blood-borne infections. The main reasons for these changes were: the HIV pandemic; the relatively high incidence of hepatitis B infections among health care workers compared with the general population; and the recognition of the rights of health care workers to occupational safety. The most critical point of this system is that staff must change their gloves for each patient. Wearing one pair of gloves all day long will protect the health care workers themselves, but may transmit infectious agents among patients. Prominent notices should call the attention of staff to the vital importance of changing gloves between patients.

Isolation at the source of infection

The aim of the interruption of the transmission of the infectious agent at the source is to localize the infection. This is achieved by:

* decontamination of the human and/or inanimate source
* physical separation of a human source using barriers.

Decontamination aims to remove or to kill the infectious agents in the source and/or within the mode of transmission (see Figure 5.1, page 117). Methods of decontamination are:

* inanimate source:
  - cleaning:
    ○ dry
    ○ wet
  - disinfection:
    ○ sterilization (complete disinfection)
    ○ selective disinfection
* human source:
  - cleaning
  - selective disinfection:
    ○ skin:
      □ skin disinfection at the site of invasive procedures
      □ hand disinfection
      □ whole-body disinfection
    ○ mucosa

    – antibiotic treatment:
       ◦ topical
       ◦ systemic.

The effect of decontamination depends on the method used, on the initial amount of the micro-organism, and on the resistance of the micro-organism. This is expressed as the reduction of the micro-organism under the defined conditions of the decontaminating method, per unit of time.

The choice of decontamination method depends on the level of the *risk of clinical infection*. On this basis, the hospital environment may be classified as:

- high risk – critical instruments that penetrate sterile tissues or blood vessels, or have contact with mucosa (surgical items, endoscopes, syringes, needles, catheters, etc.) even if contaminated initially with microbes with low virulence. These items should be free of any kind of viable micro-organisms.
- intermediate risk – semi-critical items that have direct contact with intact skin (bedclothes, stethoscope, blood pressure cuffs). Here, pathogenic microbes causing infectious diseases of the skin, or able to transmit other potential pathogens, should be absent.
- low risk – non-critical items that do not have direct contact with people, and especially with patients (e.g. walls, floor). But if *Bacillus anthracis* – a very dangerous infectious disease – is found on the walls or floor the environment cannot then be described as 'low risk'. Low risk items should be free of absolute pathogen.

In the original classification, items in contact with mucous membranes were regarded as semi-critical, and items in contact with intact skin as non-critical. However, there is no guarantee that the mucous membranes remain intact (i.e. are not injured) during endoscopy and other medical procedures, and so such items should be classified as 'high risk'. There is evidence that infections with clinical consequences have followed endoscopic procedures (O'Connor and Axon, 1983; Alvarado et al., 1991). Items in direct contact with skin may transmit fungi or other pathogenic bacteria, causing clinical infection, which also confirms the need to reclassify such procedures. The classification of the hospital environment for immuno-compromised patients (who have, for example, received bone marrow transplantation or other organ transplants) needs refinement.

Cleaning

Cleaning removes the microbes by physical (mechanical or dissolving) and/or chemical (detergent) methods. But microbes removed by cleaning may survive to fight another day. The decontaminating effect of cleaning is such that there is no guarantee of the complete removal of microbes. Therefore, cleaning must be used only for items with a low risk of infection and not for pre-cleaning items with an intermediate or high risk of infection, before disinfection and sterilization.

Dry cleaning removes only the superficial dust, and the critical point is that it raises clouds of dust in the air. This can be quite dangerous as *Mycobacteria* and other micro-organisms can survive in the dust. A dry cloth or vacuum cleaning is normally used to remove dust. These methods should be avoided in health care settings. Despite the lack of firm evidence that carpets contribute to a higher incidence of HAI, it is not recommended that such surfaces, which can be cleaned only by a dry method, be used in hospital and health care settings.

Wet cleaning with a solvent (such as water, or water plus detergent) dissolves the organic substance and dust with micro-organisms without raising a cloud of dust. It is used for cleaning items with a low risk of infection, such as everyday cleaning of floors and walls. Despite professional criticism of this method, it is also licensed for pre-cleaning of items (medical instruments) before disinfection or sterilization. The most common domestic method of wet cleaning is hand washing with soap, but this is not allowed in hospitals because nosocomial pathogens may be transmitted via the bar of soap.

If the dissolving substance is contaminated with an infectious agent, then the item being 'cleaned' will be contaminated with this agent. Hence the requirement is that the dissolving substance should be free of any infectious agent. However, in practice it is impossible to use sterile dissolving substances for cleaning every time. The most frequently used solvent – tap water – may contain different bacteria (*Pseudomonas, Acinetobacter, Serratia, Escherichia, Proteus, Klebsiella, Legionella,* etc.) from the water mains or from the external surface of the tap.

Disinfection

Disinfection is defined as the killing of microbes in both the animate and inanimate environment. The resistance of micro-organisms is not uniform against different disinfectant agents. Complete disinfection (= sterilization) means that the disinfectant (sterilant) kills even the most resistant infectious agent on the resistance scale. Disinfection is said to be incomplete if the disinfectant does not kill every type of micro-organism (selective killing).

Two main types of disinfection are used:

- physical
- chemical.

The essence of both types of disinfection is the use of physical energy or chemical molecules to kill the living organism by means of the denaturation of the essential structural and enzyme proteins and/or fracturing the nucleic acid (DNA or RNA) sequence of the genetic substance of the microbe. The effect of killing by physical means depends on the amount of physical energy (temperature, dose of radiation or other physical agent) and on the time of exposure. The effect of killing by chemicals depends mainly on the toxicity, on the amount of disinfectant, and also on the exposure time. Both type of disinfection are influenced by the type of microbial contamination, which determines the resistance against the disinfection method, and by the presence of organic substances. Temperature alters the effectiveness of chemical disinfection. An increase in temperature reduces the time required to kill by chemical disinfectant.

Hundreds of chemical molecules have been found to have a disinfectant effect. They belong to the following groups: aldehyde, alcohol, alkylamine, chlorine, iodine, glycoles, guanidine, akaline, peroxide, phenol, inorganic acids, organic acids.

Several indicator micro-organisms are used to measure the degree of resistance to chemical disinfectants. Figure 5.2 shows the degree of resistance of various micro-organisms. There is necessarily some overlap between the grades of resistance.

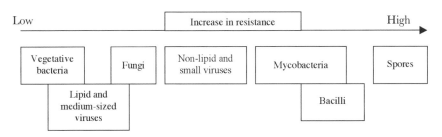

Figure 5.2. Resistance scale of the groups of indicator micro-organisms against chemical disinfectants.

Prions have not been included in the scale, as so far their resistance to disinfectants has not been assessed completely (Brown et al., 2001).

If a disinfectant has a killing effect then it carries the suffix '-cide', but if it only inhibits the growth of micro-organisms then it is labelled as '-static', and has limited disinfection effect. Ideally a disinfectant would have a 'cide' effect against all micro-organisms rather than a 'static' effect, but in practice this is impossible. Because many disinfectants kill micro-organisms selectively, there has been an attempt to classify them into three main groups according to the level of disinfection:

- high level (killing all microbes, including *Mycobacteria* and spores
- intermediate level – killing all microbes, but with limited action against spores and some nonlipid and small viruses
- low level – killing only vegetative bacteria, lipid and medium-sized viruses, and limited action against fungi.

Some overlap also occurs in this classification, but this characterization is important for comparing the anti-microbial spectrum of all the disinfectants. If the aim of the disinfection is to kill all possible micro-organisms except spores and *Mycobacteria*, even then disinfectants with tuberculocide effect (killing *Mycobacteria*) are recommended in order to increase the margin of safety.

Micro-organisms do not usually occur alone in the environment – they are surrounded by organic matter. The amount of organic matter depends on the degree of moisture. Organic matter contains proteins, lipids and other substances that protect the micro-organisms from the disinfectant, so reducing the killing effect. Hence, dissolving the organic matter is necessary for all types of disinfection. As the organic matter reduces the killing effect of disinfectant, the best disinfectants are those that can dissolve the organic matter and kill microbes at the same time. However, most chemical disinfectants cannot do this alone, and require the addition of detergent to the disinfectant agent. Compatibility of the detergent and disinfectant is an important issue. If the disinfectant agent does not have a compatible detergent, pre-cleaning is required before using the disinfectant in order first to remove the organic matter. Cleaning and disinfection in separate phases must be used only for floors and walls. Careful rinsing is then needed before the disinfectant is applied.

In practice, the term 'disinfection' is used for incomplete or selective types, while the term 'sterilization' is used for complete disinfection. Professionally, the distinction between these two terms should be maintained.

Complete disinfection (sterilization)

Sterilization, or complete disinfection, is the process whereby items become sterile by killing all the living organisms.

Sterilization in medicine began with the improvement of surgical asepsis in order to develop sterilization methods that kill any potential infectious agent occurring on Earth, without damaging the sterilized items.

The uses of sterilization are:

- decontamination of high-risk items used for procedures on the human body, preventing procedure-associated infections if there is a high risk of developing infectious disease (see Figure 5.3)
- within the pharmaceutical industry
- decontamination of infectious waste
- other non-medical uses (preservation of food, etc.).

Sterility means the absence of any living organism in any form. The term 'sterile' is an absolute term, but in practice it is limited by our ability to *detect* micro-organisms.

Sterilization cycle is defined as the set of all the parameters of a sterilizing agent in order to achieve sterility. The same sterilant may have different parameters, which defines different cycles.

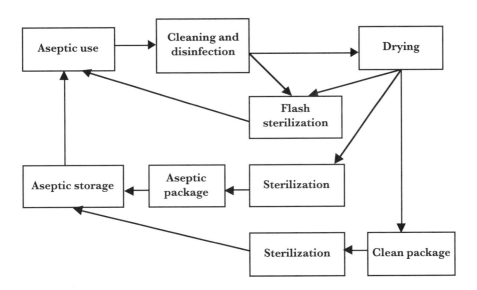

Figure 5.3. Process of aseptic use of reusable medical instruments.

Load is defined as an article with its own special characteristics in terms of sterilization. There are different loads: surgical instrument, solution for parenteral use, textile, implantable device, etc. Combination of different parameters with different load configurations results in different types of sterilization processes.

Batch is the content that is treated in a single sterilization cycle.

Sterilization process is a broader term than sterilization cycle as it consists of other essential conditions (cleaning, packing, storage) required to achieve sterility. The sterilization processes, including the load configuration plus sterilization cycle, should be validated and certified individually by a competent authority.

It is important to find the most resistant micro-organism (test organism = bio-indicator) for the specified method in order to define the parameters of sterilization regarding the safety level and quality assurance. It is based on the assumption that if the sterilization method with certain defined parameters kills the most resistant germ then the sterilized item will probably be free of all living micro-organisms. As a result of microbiological research and medical observation, strains of genera of *Bacillus* have been accepted internationally as the most resistant and are therefore chosen as test organisms for different sterilization methods (European Directorate for the Quality of Medicines, 1997; United States Pharmacopeial Convention, 2000). However, the latest research has shown that *prions*, being infective proteins – among them a prion causing Creutzfeldt-Jakob disease in humans – surpass the *Bacillus* in heat resistance, which may result in a potential hazard of prion infection for humans after the regular sterilization process with heat (WHO, 1999). Prions may also show unusually high resistance to ionizing radiation (Gibbs et al., 1978).

D value (decimal reduction value) is used to express mathematically the resistance of a micro-organism against a physical or chemical agent, which is equal to a parameter of the agent (duration – usually in minutes, or the absorbed dose) required to reduce the microbial population by 90% or 1 log cycle (i.e. one microbe in ten survives). For example, the minimum D value for *Bacillus stearothermophilus* is equal to 1.5 minutes in saturated steam at 121°C.

Lethality input (*LI*) is the amount of energy absorbed during the treatment process expressed relative to the D value, taking the resistance of the known test organism as a standard. For example, if the treatment with saturated steam lasts for 15 minutes at 121° C, the lethality input is equal to 10D

$(15/1.5 = 10)$ taking the survival of *Bacillus stearothermophilus* as standard with a D value of 1.5 minutes.

Inactivation of micro-organisms by physical and chemical agents follows an exponential law, which means that there is always a statistical probability of microbial survival of the sterilization.

The *sterility assurance level (SAL)* of a sterilization process is the degree of assurance expressed as a probability of a non-sterile item remaining in the population of the items undergoing a sterilization process. A 10^{-3} probability of survival means that there is one chance in one thousand that viable organisms are present on the sterilized item, i.e. one test in 1000 will yield a positive result. A SAL of 10^{-6} or greater is generally accepted for terminally sterilized items, i.e. one chance or less in one million (European Directorate for the Quality of Medicines, 1997; United States Pharmacopeial Convention, 2000).

The *overkill approach* is so called if the duration of the sterilization process exceeds the critical time required to achieve a SAL greater than 10^{-6}. However, for many items it may not be feasible to achieve the overkill approach – for example with heat-sensitive items – in which case the individual biological burden should be estimated by the SAL using parameters other than the standard cycle.

The SAL and the parameters required for the overkill approach are estimated according to the following criteria:

• the initial number of micro-organisms present on the item
• the resistance of the micro-organisms contaminating the item compared with the resistance of the standard test organism
• the D-value of the standard test organism at the chosen parameters
• the environment of the sterilization process influencing the D-value.

For example, if the required SAL is 10^{-6}, the resistance of the micro-organism against the saturated steam at 121°C is $D_{121} = 3$ minutes, and if the initial microbial burden is 100 microbes/treated unit, then 27 minutes are needed to reach the estimated probability of SAL (see Table 5.1).

As the survival of whole cell microbes can be counted only in integers, $D_{121} = 6$ minutes or 2D of the lethality input yields a microbial burden of 1 (10^0 estimated) and the additional 21 minutes, i.e. 6D, yields a calculated survival probability (see Table 5.1).

The critical issue is knowing the resistance of the expected natural microbial burden relative to the test organism. Thus it is important to demonstrate

Table 5.1. Estimated probability of the sterility assurance level (SAL)

Treatment time in minutes	Microbial count	Probability of SAL
0	100	non-sterile
3	10	non-sterile
6	1	non-sterile
9	0.1	1 non-sterile in 10 (10^1)
12	0.01	1 non-sterile in 100 (10^2)
18	0.001	1 non-sterile in 1000 (10^3)
21	0.0001	1 non-sterile in 10,000 (10^4)
24	0.00001	1 non-sterile in 100,000 (10^5)
27	0.000001	1 non-sterile in 1,000,000 (10^6)

D_{121} of the test organism = 3 minutes.

during validation that the sterilization process is capable of removing the infectious agents with even greater resistance than the test organism, giving priority to the D-values, the SAL, the magnitude of the initial natural contamination on the item, and the amount of the test organism.

Where the viable units of an infectious agent are measured on another scale, rather than by 'count', additional validation is needed. This is the case if the product is contaminated by prions that can be inactivated with saturated steam of 134°C for 60 minutes (WHO, 1999). In case of pyrogen challenge, further validation is needed by measuring the level of the inactivation of endotoxins on/in the sterilized item after contamination of the item with a known quantity of bacterial endotoxin.

The essential requirement for all types of sterilization is that all parts of the item should be in contact with the sterilizing agent. However, it should be taken into account that access to the sterilant is not uniform at each point of the item. The critical issue is the presence of so-called 'cold points', which have no contact with the sterilant, thus remaining non-sterile. It is therefore important to determine the minimum lethality input to ensure that the load at each point (even at all the cold points) will consistently receive treatment exceeding the minimum SAL.

Methods of sterilization:

- physical:
  - heat:
    - boiling
    - burning or incineration

- ○ saturated steam
- ○ dry heat
- − ionizing radiation:
  - ○ gamma rays
  - ○ microwaves
  - ○ X-rays
  - ○ electrons
- − ultraviolet (UV) radiation
- − filtration
- chemical:
  - − gas-vapour sterilants:
    - ○ ethylene oxide (EO) gas
    - ○ formaldehyde vapour
    - ○ vapour-phase hydrogen peroxide
    - ○ plasma gas
  - − chlorine dioxide gas
  - − ozone
  - − cold liquid sterilization:
    - ○ peracetic acid
    - ○ glutaraldehyde.

Forms of sterilization:

- industrial (food industry, space technology, etc.)
- hospital or health care settings:
  - − centralized – at a central unit
  - − decentralized – within departments
- other non-medical (tattoo studios, etc.).

Heat is the most common method of sterilization in health care owing to its relatively low cost and ease of control, with low levels of hazard to personnel and patients compared with chemical methods.

Boiling is one of the oldest methods of sterilization. The process is done at 100°C (212°F) for 30 minutes. Sodium carbonate is added in order to increase the pH of the water in an alkaline direction, which makes it easier to kill even spores. It was widely used in surgery when the boilers functioned close to operating theatres and the metal surgical instruments were used immediately. The process is now out of date, difficult to control, and the aseptic storage of boiled instruments for further use is not guaranteed, re-contamination may occur, and the contamination of water with dust is unavoidable. This method had persisted until the introduction of saturated steam and dry heat, and nowadays it is not recommended for the regular sterilization of instruments in hospitals. It may be used only in wartime or when no other methods of sterilization are available.

In abdominal surgery *hot water* is quite often used to stop capillary bleeding, promoting the coagulation of blood by heat. For this purpose hot water used to be prepared in the operating theatre by freshly boiling it on an electric or gas plate. Nowadays this has been replaced by heating pre-sterilized bottled water in a microwave oven, or in some other way.

Burning has been used as a method of sterilization since ancient and medieval times, with the fire temperature more than 300°C (572°F). It is one of the best methods to decontaminate infectious material. This method was used during outbreaks of dangerous infections like plague, burning all contaminated equipment. It is used today in hospitals for burning hospital waste and for decontamination of laboratory waste. This method is still recommended for decontamination of equipment in extremely dangerous infections (such as Lassa fever, yellow fever, plague).

Saturated steam, using the appropriate concentration of water and pressure for a defined time, is the most economical and efficient way of sterilizing instruments. It kills the living organisms by denaturation of the heat-sensitive cellular and/or soluble proteins of microbes. Because the condensation of saturated steam kills the micro-organisms, the quality of the steam is important. Dry heat is less effective than saturated steam, but if the steam is too wet it may leave the item non-sterile. Saturated steam should be the first choice of sterilization if the item is heat and moisture stable. The requirement is that all surfaces should be directly exposed to steam, with adequate steam circulation. This is achieved by the removal of air from the chamber, after which steam is introduced under pressure. Technically, there are two main types of steam sterilizer:

- the gravity displacement sterilizer – which displaces air from the chamber and loads steam by gravity
- the pre-vacuum sterilizer – which removes the air from the chamber and loads the steam by means of a vacuum pump. This is faster than gravity displacement owing to the higher speed and greater efficiency of the air removal.

Two systems are:

- the wrapped method, when items are wrapped in textile, special paper, or metallic boxes with filters, or in other packing material allowing steam penetration, while preventing recontamination during storage
- flash sterilization or emergency sterilization, when unwrapped items are to be used immediately after the sterilization.

Dry heat uses the same mechanism of action for sterilization as saturated steam. It denatures proteins but is less effective than the saturated steam, needing higher temperatures and more time to achieve the same result. Two parameters are controlled: temperature and time.

Gamma radiation achieves sterilization by the penetration of gamma rays, so destroying the genetic material. Usually cobalt-60 weapon (Co-60) is used. Gamma rays penetrate all materials, leaving no cold points. This is the best method of sterilization if the amount of energy available is adequate. However, it is available only for industrial use, as it needs strict safety regulations. Items remain sterile for two to five years, depending on the packaging and the characteristics of the item. Most disposable medical instruments are sterilized in this way.

Microwave energy has been used for sterilization since the second half of the twentieth century. It works by heating the item. The combined effect of non-thermal and thermal waves leads to destruction of the micro-organisms. It is used for flash sterilization of microbiological media.

Electrons used for sterilization are produced by an accelerator generating and focusing a high-energy electron beam. Used in industry, its penetration is less than that of gamma rays.

Ultraviolet radiation (UV) consists of electromagnetic waves which act on nucleic acids. It is produced by germicidal lamps and tubes, giving a blue-violet light that can damage the human eye. It does not penetrate and so can be used only for air and surface sterilization with direct exposure. Its effectiveness depends strongly on the intensity of the light, the distance from the source, microbial resistance to UV radiation, and the relative humidity. It is used in laboratories to avoid laboratory contamination (PCR laboratories, mycology, etc.).

Filtration is used for decontamination of liquids using membrane filters with different pore sizes, removing microbes that are physically larger than the pores. This method is used for the filtration of ethyl alcohol, which does not have a sporocidal effect, in order to remove spores.

Gas-vapour sterilants achieve their killing effect by chemical reactions inactivating the organic material of microbes, leading to their destruction. They are used for the sterilization of heat-sensitive items. Critical points for them are the gas concentration, humidity, temperature, and the carrier material. Penetration of chemicals differs according to which gas is used and the characteristics of the item. They usually act on surfaces, or on the inner surfaces of open lumens. The most vulnerable aspect is the presence of organic material that protects microbes from the gas.

Ethylene oxide (EO) has a sporocidal action due to alkylation of different organic molecules. It is considered to be a mutagen and carcinogen, so its emission should be controlled during the sterilization process and the storage of the items. Items may adsorb EO, which can be quickly removed by active aeration in an aerator after the sterilization. The passive emission of EO from items at room temperature lasts about four to 14 days or more. However, plastic and rubber items may emit EO for several days even after aeration, threatening both the patients and staff in direct contact with the item. EO is standardized in both the USA and Europe. Items should be in 'toxicological quarantine' – usually for four days if the emission is passive, or two days in the case of active aeration. Owing to its toxicity it is recommended only for those items that cannot be sterilized by other methods.

Formaldehyde vapour is the second most widely used chemical sterilant. It has a sporocidal action, denaturing proteins and destroying nucleic acid. It is also carcinogenic, and the same control measures are needed as for EO. Residues may also be detected on some items, but the aeration phase is replaced by a washout period at the end of sterilization, which reduces the duration of the emission. This is standardized in the USA and in the EU. There is no specific time for toxicological quarantine.

Vapour-phase hydrogen peroxide is a highly sporocidal agent, acting as an oxidant producing non-toxic radicals. Corrosive features (due to 30% hydrogen peroxide) and low penetration limit its use in everyday medical practice.

Plasma gas has recently been applied and standardized in the USA and the EU, and is called 'plasma sterilization'. It also works with vaporized hydrogen peroxide, which is converted into gas plasma by radio waves. The process is carried out twice. The free radicals destroy the nucleic acid, killing the microbes. Deep vacuum is needed for appropriate diffusion of the vapour, which may destroy some items. Items with lumens need special preparation with the application of a balloon containing hydrogen peroxide, which makes this method of sterilization rather complicated. Due to the non-toxic end product it is better toxicologically than EO or formaldehyde vapour – replacing them in hospitals. There is no need for toxicological quarantine.

Chlorine dioxide has been investigated for sterilization of medical equipment but has not been standardized and is not used in hospitals. It oxidizes proteins without altering the nucleic acid. Its short- and long-term effects are not well defined.

Ozone has also been investigated for sterilization. It has an oxidative effect on proteins. The process ends with the production of non-toxic substances. It has not been standardized for hospitals owing to its low penetrability and its corrosive effect on plastics and metals.

Sterilization in cold liquids is usually called 'cold sterilization' because it is carried out at room temperature. Peracetic acid and glutaraldehyde are well-standardized methods and are used widely in hospitals throughout the world (see Annexe 1 and Annexe 2).

Peracetic acid is an oxidizing agent that attacks proteins. It is sporocidal alone or in combination with hydrogen peroxide. Its use is limited to materials that can be immersed. Rinsing with sterile water is required at the end of the process to remove toxic radicals. It is not a widely used method.

Glutaraldehyde solution in 2% concentration is widely used for instruments that cannot be sterilized by heat or radiation. The exposure time is several hours depending on the sporocidal effect. It alkylates different organic molecules, killing micro-organisms. It is toxic, and proper rinsing of instruments with sterile water is essential. Packaging should be done in a sterile room in aseptic conditions (sterile gloves, coat, mask, etc.).

Quality control of sterilization

Quality control is essential for all steps in the sterilization process of items for aseptic use (cleaning, packaging, sterilization cycle, and storage).

Quality control begins with the cleaning of items. As the initial amount of microbes affects the final effect of sterilization, the items should harbour as few microbes as possible before the sterilization cycle. Items should be clean with no visible dust or any other substance on the outside or inside surface. This can be achieved with careful cleaning and preparation, without recontamination. Items should be blood-free, as prions may survive the regular standardized sterilization process, taking *Bacillus* as the test organism. Cleaning is controlled by:

- inspection of the item
- chemical detection of blood remaining on the item.

Chemical detection of blood remaining on the surface of items, especially surgical instruments, is an objective method of control in the item's preparation. Gregersen reagent can be used to detect invisible blood contamination; 0.125 g Gregersen reagent contains one part benzidine and four parts barium hyperoxide dissolved in 5 ml 50% acetic acid. The reagent should be prepared freshly and dropped on to the instrument. If the instrument is contaminated with blood the yellow-brown colour of the reagent changes to a blue-green colour within 15 minutes. Data on blood contamination of prepared items before sterilization at hospital 'A' in Hungary can be seen in Table 5.2.

Table 5.2. Percentage of surgical instruments contaminated with blood after cleaning and disinfection but before sterilization at hospital 'A', Hungary

Year	Number of instruments tested	Contaminated with blood %
1995	203	22.60
1996	521	28.02
1997	633	23.70
1998	849	17.79
1999	ND	
2000	792	18.06

ND = no data.

Packaging should be standardized according to the penetrability of the sterilant, and it should prevent recontamination of the sterilized item during storage. Different packaging systems have been developed, such as metal boxes with filters, textiles and paper. In storage the outside of the package may be contaminated with dust (and spores of anaerobic bacteria!), which can recontaminate the sterilized item when opening. The safest method is for the package to contain at least two layers in order to reduce the risk of recontamination, and to carefully open the outside layer first and then the inner layer. This is extremely important in operating theatres because the sterile gloves of the sterile nurse can also become contaminated with dust during the opening of the package. Standard sterilization processes are validated by using a specified type of package, and only such a standard package can be used. Packages other than the standard ones should be validated according to the sterilization parameters.

The sterilization cycle is controlled in order to check that the items are exposed according to the parameters of the sterilizing agent, and are made safe for use. The parameters are regulated first by national pharmacopoeia as the standard reference. In Europe, 27 countries have signed the European Pharmacopoeia Convention, adopting the European Pharmacopoeia as a compulsory document. Both the US and the European Pharmacopoeia regulate five types of sterilization (wet heat, dry heat, ionizing radiation, gas sterilization, and filtration) and the aseptic preparation of the items sterilized by one of the above-mentioned processes. Pharmacopoeias give only one set of parameters as a reference and they allow the development of other cycles of the same sterilant if they have the same effect as the reference cycle (see Table 5.3).

Alternatively, sterilization can be standardized by national standards, or by other specifications. There may be some differences in the required parameters of the same sterilant, but within the safety assurance level. Generally such differences in the required parameters can be grouped as:

- standardized cycle – exact standard values, or a range of the parameters, with defined types of load are allowed based on the interrelation of each parameter if their combined safety can be proved (see Table 5.3)
- individual parameters – parameters can be completely different from the standard fixed or ranged values because they are based on the estimated initial amount of contaminating micro-organisms and on their resistance against the sterilant for the given item, which is tested individually.

In those countries where a fixed standard or a range of the parameters only are allowed, manufacturers of medical items must take into account the parameters of the standardized cycle by modifying the item to be resistant to the sterilization cycle without suffering any damage. Where individual parameters are allowed, the manufacturers of the medical items are allowed to modify the parameters if this is necessary to achieve 'sterility' without damaging the item, but they must test and report the individual parameters of the sterilization cycle of the specified item.

Control of the sterilization cycle has two main purposes:

- for validation of the cycle during the installation qualification
- to enable users to:
  - routinely monitor the cycle
  - revalidate a previously validated cycle after major repair
  - release processed items.

Table 5.3. Summary of the main sterilization methods in hospitals

Sterilant	Organization	Technical type	Parameters			Test organism
			Temperature	Time	Other	
Wet heat	United States Pharmacopoeia	Not specified, reference condition	121 ± 1°C	5 min		*Bacillus stearothermophilus*
	European Pharmacopoeia	Not specified, reference condition	121°C	15 min		*Bacillus stearothermophilus*
	American National Standard	Gravity displacement	132–135°C (270–275°F) 121–123°C (250–254°F)	10–25 min 15–30 min		*Bacillus stearothermophilus* *Bacillus stearothermophilus*
		Steam-flush, gravity displacement	132°C (270°F)	3–10 min		*Bacillus stearothermophilus*
		Steam-flush, prevacuum displacement	132–135°C (270–275°F)	3–4 min		*Bacillus stearothermophilus*
		Steam-flush, pressure-pulse cycles	141–144°C (285–291°F) 132–135°C (270–275°F) 121–123°C (250–254°F)	2 min 3–4 min 20 min		*Bacillus stearothermophilus* *Bacillus stearothermophilus* *Bacillus stearothermophilus*
Dry heat	United States Pharmacopoeia	Not specified, reference condition	250 ± 15°C	No exact value		*Bacillus subtilis*
	European Pharmacopoeia	Not specified, reference condition	160°C	120 min		*Bacillus subtilis varians niger*
	American National Standard	Static air type	160°C (320°F) or higher	No exact value		Not specified, SAL must be 10⁻⁶ probability of surviving
		Forced air type	160°C (320°F) or higher	No exact value		Not specified, SAL must be 10⁻⁶ probability of surviving

Method	Standard		Temperature	Time	Concentration	Biological indicator
Ethylene oxide vapour	United States Pharmacopoeia	Not specified	No exact values	No exact value	No values	Bacillus subtilis
	European Pharmacopoeia	Not specified, reference condition	54°C (129°F)	60 min	EO concentration: 600 mg/L, relative humidity: 60%	Bacillus subtilis varians niger
	American National Standard	Not specified	37–63°C (99–145°F)	60–360 min	EO concentration: 450–1200 mg/L, relative humidity: 40–80%	Bacillus subtilis
Formaldehyde vapour	United States Pharmacopoeia	Not specified	No exact values	No exact values	No exact value	Not specified
	European Pharmacopoeia	Not specified	No exact values	No exact values	No exact value	Bacillus subtilis varians niger
	American National Standard	Formaldehyde/alcohol mixture, table top	132°C (270°F)	20min	No exact value	Not specified
Liquid peracetic acid	European Pharmacopoeia	Not specified	No exact values	No exact values	No exact value	Bacillus stearothermophilus
	Food and Drug Administration, USA	Not specified	50–56°C (122–133°F)	12 min	35% liquid peracetic acid is diluted to its 0.2% use dilution	Not specified
	American National Standard	Not specified	20°C (68°F)	8 hours	1% hydrogen peroxide and 0.08% peracetic acid	Not specified
Glutaraldehyde	Food and Drug Administration, USA	Not specified	20–25°C (68–77°F)	10 hours	2.4-3.4% of glutaraldehyde depending on the product formulation	Not specified
Gas plasma	Food and Drug Administration, USA	Not specified	50°C (122°F)	75 min	No exact value	Not specified

Control of sterilization is achieved in three ways, regardless of its purpose, by means of:

- technical control
- chemical indicators
- biological tests.

Technical control involves recording all the technical parameters of the sterilization cycle. It can be achieved:

- manually, by checking and writing down the parameters from the read-out
- mechanically, with graphs and charts recorded automatically by the sterilizer.

If the recorded parameters do not correspond to the standard or licensed individual ones, then the item should be classified as non-safe and must not be used until after re-sterilization with appropriate parameters. Each batch or load should be controlled technically. In practice, the batch number and date of sterilization are very important, to identify the items if there is discovered to be a cluster of infections after using items with the same batch number.

Chemical indicators contain chemical reagents, and the colour of the indicator changes as a result of exposure to the sterilants. They are used, together with the technical data, to control parameters. Several indicators have been developed. These are classified as:

- uni-parametric
- multi-parametric:
  - safety indicators
  - process indicators
  - Bowie Dick indicator.

Uni-parametric chemical indicators were the first to be introduced. They give information about only one parameter of the sterilization process by changing colour. For example, if the autoclave achieves the required temperature – even for only one second – the colour of the chemical indicator is changed. Uni-parametric indicators are appropriate only for distinguishing processed items from non-processed items, because they do not measure all the parameters of the sterilization cycle. Alone, they cannot be accepted for safety. Indicators of this type must be stuck on the outside of the package. Users must be able to distinguish this type of indicator from other types. However, the outside indicator may become lost.

Multi-parametric chemical indicators measure more than one parameter of sterilization. *Safety indicators* measure all the parameters of the sterilization process at the same time, and can be used for safety purposes. Safety indicators show whether the item is safe or not. However, an appropriate colour change does not necessarily mean that the item is sterile; it means only that all parameters of the sterilization process were adequate in the chamber. *Process indicators* are more complex as they measure separately the parameters on different points (dots) of the indicator. They are used to discover which, if any, parameter of the sterilization process is not adequate. Among the different types, some indicators measure only two parameters, for example temperature and time in the autoclave (two-parametric process indicators) while others measure all parameters (temperature, time and pressure in the autoclave). If the process indicator can measure each parameter at the same time it can be used as a safety indicator as well. Multi-parametric indicators increase the probability of safety, and they should be put in each package of every load.

The *Bowie Dick indicator* (or an equivalent) tests the steam penetration in pre-vacuum and vacuum pulsing sterilizers by removal of the air from the empty or loaded chamber, or by detecting the presence of an air leak. It is recommended for use once a day and after major repairs.

Biological tests are used to detect whether the parameters of the sterilizing agent are adequate to achieve sterility. They indicate whether the sterilization process *as a whole* is safely within the sterility assurance level. They do not provide information on which parameter of the process is inadequate.

Biological testing may be achieved by two methods:

- biological indicators
- sterility testing.

Biological indicators consist of a standardized, defined amount of viable micro-organism (the test organism) with a known resistance (D value) to the type of sterilization (see Table 5.3). If the parameters are adequate during the sterilization cycle the test organism is killed and regrowth does not occur on an appropriate medium. However, a negative biological indicator – i.e. no regrowth – does not prove that the items in the load are sterile. A negative indicator gives only a probabilistic indication of whether the item is safe or not. Similarly, a positive indicator – regrowth – does not mean that the item is not sterile, but as the probability of safety cannot be estimated, the items cannot be used. The sterilization process in this case should be rechecked, and items may be used only if the repeated results are negative. The biological indicator does not replace the mechanical and chemical controls, but together with them it increases the safety level of sterilization. The golden rule is: there is no absolute guarantee that the sterilized item is sterile.

Repeated testing of the sterilization cycle with biological indicators by the user is essentially a revalidation of the sterilization process by the user. A user's load may differ from the load used for biological validation of the standard cycle in the licensing procedure, which is not permitted but may occur in practice. Users should be familiar with the concept of D values and SAL, and all the circumstances of each biological testing should be recorded to evaluate the appropriateness of the revalidation. Manufacturers of biological indicators must label the indicator with essential information on:

- the type of bio-indicator, i.e. the exact name of the test organism
- the range of the viable count per carrier of the bio-indicator
- the D value
- survival and killing times.

Sterility tests use a culture technique, or other detection method, by taking samples direct from the surface of the sterilized item or by inserting the item into a growth medium. This is the final step in the control of the sterilization cycle, and it is also used to control storage (see below). It should be emphasized that the verification of sterility is limited by our detection methods, and that an absence of detected micro-organisms does not mean that the item is sterile. A sterility test is not an alternative to a bioindicator.

Storage is the final step in the quality control of sterilized items. The packages should be stored in dust-free conditions at moderate humidity and at room temperature in order to avoid damage and recontamination. It is important to check the expiry date. Items must not be used if they become wet, moist or beyond the expiry date, because sterility is not then guaranteed.

Routine monitoring of each cycle should be done by using technical and chemical indicators, as these give immediate information about the parameters, and the possible safety of the load. The frequency of routine monitoring by bio-indicators of the genera of *Bacillus* differs among the recommendations of different organizations (see Table 5.4). However, any technical failure, undetectable by technical control or chemical indicator, may still be caught with the biological indicator. In routine monitoring, if a test shows a positive result the items released since the last negative biological monitoring test are recalled immediately. The less frequent the routine biological monitoring the greater the risk of missing technical failures and thereby releasing non-sterile items. In terms of high quality control, it is hardly acceptable to monitor sterilization cycles biologically only once in three or six months, as suggested by the Hungarian Public Health Office (see Table 5.4).

Whether an item is safe to release is a decision that should be based on the results of the control of all the stages in the sterilization process (cleaning, package, sterilization cycle, storage). The decision should be made carefully considering all the circumstances. However, in practice release often happens without regard to the results of biological tests, giving different types of release:

- parametric release
- release by technical and chemical indicator
- release by biological indicator
- release after sterility testing.

Parametric release occurs if the sterilized items are available for immediate use if the parameters of the sterilization cycle are deemed appropriate by technical control. However, parametric release of the sterilized item is a critical issue. For maximum safety it is desirable that items are released only after total control with biological testing by bio-indicators, and by sterility testing of a representative sample of the batch sterilized in one cycle. However, keeping the items in biological quarantine – waiting for the result of biological tests – may increase the number of items stocked, which is not always feasible in practice. The European Pharmacopoeia allows parametric release after validated terminal sterilization if a competent authority approves, while the US Pharmacopoeia does not regulate it.

Release by technical and chemical indicator is done after technical control together with appropriate results from a chemical indicator. Neither the US nor European Pharmacopoeia regulates release after technical and chemical control; it is at the user's decision. However, in practice this type of release is the most common. It is advisable to validate each batch of chemical indicators by biological test using bio-indicators.

Table 5.4. Recommended frequency of biological monitoring of sterilization processes in hospitals

Reference	Use of biological indicators generally	Regular routine biological monitoring						Biological monitoring of implant devices	Quarantine until the result of biological test is known
		Wet steam	Dry heat	Ethylene oxide	Formaldehyde vapour	Peracetic acid			
Association for the Advancement of Medical Instrumentation (AAMI)	Should be for qualification, for installation and periodically thereafter	At least weekly, but preferably daily	Regularly, but not specified	Should be at each cycle	No recommendation	No recommendation	Should be at each load	Whenever possible
Association of Operating Room Nurses (AORN)	Compulsory at regular intervals and after installation, repair, redesign, or relocation	Should be at least weekly and preferably daily	Should be at least once per week for table top design	Should be at every load	No recommendation	Should be at least weekly and preferably daily	Should be at each load	When possible, for implant devices
American Hospital Association	Should be at regular intervals, additionally when the process is in question	At least once a day	Should be once a day	Should be used preferably at every load	No recommendation	No recommendation	Every load should be	Should be until the testing results are known
Centers for Disease Control and Prevention (CDC), Atlanta	Should be monitored	At least weekly	At least weekly	At least weekly	At least weekly	At least weekly	Every load should be	Should not be used until negative spore test at 48 hours
Hungarian Public Health Office	Compulsory after installation, major repair, and regularly	At least every six months	At least every six months	At least every six months	At least every three months	No recommendation	No recommendation	No recommendation

Release by biological indicator means the batch must be in biological quarantine until negative results are obtained with the bio-indicator test. For implantable devices some organizations recommend this type of release (see Table 5.4).

Release after sterility testing is allowed after negative results, regulated by the US and European Pharmacopoeias for medical products with a high risk of infection (parenteral drugs, etc.). An adequate number of samples of articles in the batch must be tested in order to obtain a statistically acceptable result, but even this may be inadequate if a small proportion of articles in the batch reveal microbial contamination. However, it is accepted because it is not possible to test all the articles in the batch. So it is always better to do sterility testing with the bio-indicator test.

Selective disinfection

Despite selective killing, incomplete disinfection is widely practised in hospitals, which is a compromise for several reasons:

- Most of the vegetative bacteria and viruses causing HAI can be killed by even a selective disinfectant.
- The number of micro-organisms can be reduced below the disease dose, which does not prevent the transmission of the infectious agent, but which may prevent the development of infectious disease.
- It is difficult to develop a disinfectant that kills every type of micro-organism while keeping the host tissues alive if the aim is to decontaminate the human body as a source or as a vehicle of the transmission of infection.
- Selective chemical disinfectants at lower concentrations may have less toxicity, which is important for the occupational safety of staff working with the disinfectant.

The same two main methods (physical and chemical) are used for selective disinfection as for sterilization, but the difference is in the dose and the duration of the exposure, which are usually less than are required to kill all micro-organisms, which is the case in sterilization.

Wet heat is also used for disinfection as for sterilization, but the temperature is usually lower than 100°C (212°F). It is widely used, for example, to decontaminate clothes infested with ectoparasites such as lice.

Ultrasound uses a low-kilohertz frequency range to deactivate micro-organisms in aqueous suspension. The effect is known as transient cavitation. Ultrasonic cleaners and sonicators are used mainly for cleaning and selective disinfection. Sterility with chemicals may be achieved, but this has not been standardized.

Chemical disinfection is the most widely used method of selective decontamination of both the inanimate environment and the animate (human body). Usually a low or intermediate level of disinfection is used, but in rare situations a high level is required.

Disinfection of the inanimate environment

As the inanimate environment can serve as the source or the vehicle of the transmission of an infectious agent, it is necessary to decontaminate it in order to control the infection. In health care settings the next parts of the inanimate environment that need decontamination are:

- surfaces
- textiles
- equipment
- water
- air.

Surfaces are contaminated with dust that may harbour *Mycobacteria* or spores of anaerobic bacteria or other infectious agents that contaminate surfaces in other ways, for example discharges (vomit, skin squama, blood, etc.). Surfaces always contain moist and organic matter protecting the micro-organisms. The principles are the same as mentioned above, and if possible the same disinfectant should be used, incorporating both cleaning and disinfecting effects in one phase. While surfaces of general wards or intensive care units carry a low risk of infection, in operating rooms dust may contaminate the sterile instruments, thereby transmitting infectious agents. This is why surfaces in operating rooms are classified as of intermediate risk, or even high risk, of infection even though they do not have direct contact with the patient (apart from the operating table). Also, surfaces in operating rooms are contam-inated much more frequently with blood and other discharges.

The potential hazard of the surfaces and the types and amounts of moisture define the types of surface disinfection, which can be classified as:

- surfaces having a low risk of infection:
  - regular everyday cleaning-disinfection

  – ad hoc disinfection – if the surface is contaminated with a discharge
- surfaces in high-risk areas of infection (operating rooms, angiography areas, etc.).

Regular everyday surface disinfection in low-risk areas is adequate by means of wet cleaning with a low level of disinfection because the aim is mainly to clean the surface and make it dust free. The frequency is undefined, but at least three times per day is recommended in areas where there are patients, or even more often if the moisture is substantial and can be removed only by more frequent cleaning.

  Ad hoc surface disinfection should be done whenever the surface becomes contaminated with any discharges. In this case a high level of disinfection is required, with tuberculocide effect, in order to kill all the possible micro-organisms safely, allowing for a lower resistance to the disinfectant than to *Mycobacteria*.

  Surfaces of high-risk areas should be disinfected with a high-level disinfectant (tuberculocide effect) because the risk of the infection is high if these surfaces are damp or dusty. In operating theatres the surfaces get soiled during almost every operation. Disinfection should be done immediately after each operation (it is, of course, prohibited to do this during operations). Disinfectants spread on the surface have a residual effect of decontaminating the dust that settles on the surface, and prevents the raising of clouds of dust. Other areas in hospitals with a similar high risk of infection should be treated like operating theatres.

  Textiles can be a dangerous source of infectious agents, thus their decontamination is very important. This can be done by thermo-disinfection, chemo-disinfection or chemo-thermo-disinfection in the laundry. Careful collection and separation is essential when staff work with soiled textiles.

  Equipment used in hospitals is either:

- disposable equipment, or
- reusable.

Disposable equipment is produced for single use and is often made of plastic, which can be damaged by frequent cleaning and disinfection. Its advantage is that single use removes the possibility of transmission of infectious agents between patients. However, the cost may be substantial, which often forces hospitals to reuse such equipment after cleaning, disinfecting and even after sterilizing, but this is not recommended because:

- there is no guarantee that disposable equipment can be disinfected or cleaned with complete removal of blood or other discharges
- damage may occur during cleaning and disinfection or even sterilization, which may cause harm to patients.

Professionally, there are no circumstances in which disposable equipment may be reused. Hospitals that reuse disposable equipment argue that they have no evidence that reuse of disposable equipment after sterilization or disinfection will spread any microbes, or harm patients in any other way. However, this is an ethical issue, and even one case of HAI due to the reuse of disposable equipment cannot be allowed. The lack of evidence of any possible infection after reuse of disposable equipment is due to the absence of scientific studies, but ethically it is not permitted to implement such research and risk the life of any patient. The solution is to use available reusable equipment where, on a cost/benefit basis, it can replace disposable equipment.

Infectious waste consists of disposable equipment that has been used for health care and should be assumed to be contaminated with infectious agents. It should be collected separately in special bags or containers, labelled, and then decontaminated by burning or by other methods.

Reusable equipment is designed for multiple use, with regular decontamination between each use without damage, and with a high probability of successful decontamination by the standard methods. It is the responsibility of the manufacturers of reusable equipment to provide information to the user about the correct method of decontamination of the item. It is strongly recommended that the disinfection and cleaning be done in one operation, both dissolving organic material and killing micro-organisms at the same time.

Disinfection and cleaning of reusable equipment should be done in a separate room (called a *disinfecting room*) set aside specially for the purpose, thereby avoiding unnecessary contamination of the environment, particularly of clean and sterile equipment. Technically two main methods are applied:

- manual
- washer:
  - mechanical
  - ultrasound.

Whichever technique is used, it is most important to immerse the soiled equipment in a cleaning-disinfecting solution immediately after use at the nearest site, for the following reasons:

- Human blood and other discharges have a highly corrosive effect, damaging metallic equipment, and should therefore be dealt with immediately.
- If blood and other discharges dry on the equipment they cannot easily be removed, which will entail a longer process, and may even require repetition of the disinfecting process.
- Injuries from sharp soiled instruments may occur, exposing staff to the most dangerous hazards of infection with blood-borne pathogens (hepatitis B and C, HIV, prions, etc.). This risk can be reduced if the transport of soiled instruments is delayed until after immersion for the required time in the decontamination fluid.

Occupational biohazard requires the wearing of strong gloves, protective goggles, a coat, and a mask if the disinfection is done manually, because aerosols may infect the staff. Gloves and coat are recommended when working with a washer. Staff should not count or sort soiled equipment because injuries happen more frequently during these procedures.

Water is disinfected for drinking and for other uses where clean and safe water is required. Hospitals usually have a centralized tap-water supply, but local disinfection of water may also be needed, for example, in swimming pools at health care rehabilitation centres to prevent infections being transmitted via the water. Swimming pools may transmit adenoviruses, causing epidemic conjunctival fever, *Pseudomonas aeruginosa*, folliculitis on the skin, and even infectious agents spread by the faecal–oral route (see Chapters 1 and 3).

Chlorine and ozone are most frequently used for the disinfection of water, but they have no cleaning effect and their effectiveness may be decreased by impurities in the water. Cleaning the water is required in the first phase, before disinfection, and this is done by mechanical filtering. The commonest way is by the use of sand filters, adding aluminium sulphate to promote coagulation of the soil. In the second phase, the disinfectant is added to the mechanically cleaned water to kill any micro-organisms remaining after filtration.

Air disinfection is important if an infectious agent is transmitted by air. This can be done only in an enclosed space if it is to be effective. Disinfection of the air is very important in operating theatres because air containing dust can contaminate sterile instruments with micro-organisms, resulting in a high risk of surgical wound infections. Air disinfection may be done by:

* chemicals
* physical methods.

Chemical air disinfection can be done with formaldehyde vapour or gas, or with other gases. However, formaldehyde is being phased out because of its toxicity. Rooms disinfected by this method must be made airtight for up to 24 hours. Formaldehyde has the advantage that surfaces also become disinfected at the same time, but it is advisable to avoid chemical disinfection of the air in hospitals.

Physical air disinfection may be achieved in two ways:

* by natural airing
* by artificial air conditioning.

Airing dilutes the dust and micro-organisms in the air by opening windows, which causes air movement (wind) due to differences of temperature and pressure between the two spaces. The bigger the difference in the temperature and pressure between the two spaces, the greater the speed of the airflow. It is efficient if the air blowing into the room is clean and fresh; if not it will pollute the air of the room. This method is common in dwelling houses, where the aim is also to replace the used air (containing higher levels of carbon dioxide) with fresh air from outside. However, its effect is uncertain in the prevention of transmission of infectious agents because the cleanliness of the 'fresh' air is beyond human control. Nevertheless, it is thought that respiratory illnesses are commonest in winter because of inadequate airing of rooms.

Air conditioning is done artificially using the same principles as airing, but the cleanness and rate of change of the air are known because they are controlled by a technical system. In addition, there is no toxic hazard comparable with formaldehyde. Air is taken from outside the building, or by recirculating partially used air, and it is then cleaned of dust by coarse filters. Finally it is disinfected by physical methods, using bacterial filters with an appropriate pore size (usually 0.2 μm) to remove micro-organisms. The air may also be warmed and cooled at this stage. Cleaned and filtered air is loaded under pressure and the air is ducted into occupied areas, while stale air is drawn out to be cleansed of dust and micro-organisms. The degree of the cleanness of the air in the room depends on the quality of the air from the air-conditioner and the rate of change of the air in the room. It is advisable to change the air 20 times per hour to decrease substantially the quantity of dust and micro-organisms in the air of a closed room.

Air conditioning is the commonest way to remove the skin scales (harbouring skin flora) of the operating team from the air, preventing surgical wound contamination.

The commonest infection that is *transmitted* by air conditioners is legionellosis, caused by *Legionella pneumophila* (Eickhoff, 1979). Its reservoir is the soil, which contaminates the water in the cooling tower of the air conditioner, so becoming the source of the infection. The infectious agent passes through the air ducts into rooms if bacterial filters are omitted from the system or if they are faulty, inducing respiratory tract infection. Regular checks, microbiological monitoring and disinfection of the water tower of the cooling system is essential, with appropriate bacterial filters in the system to prevent legionellosis and other infections.

Skin disinfection

The aim of skin disinfection is to kill or remove micro-organisms from the skin, as a possible endogenous source of infection, or when the infectious agent is transmitted by hand contact. Normally the skin is always contaminated with different micro-organisms, called skin flora, which are grouped into:

* resident flora
* transient flora.

Resident flora multiply in both the deep and superficial skin layers, surviving for a long time. It is difficult to remove microbes from the deep layers by cleaning, but disinfectants capable of penetrating there may reduce the number of microbes by killing them or inhibiting their growth. Resident flora consist mainly of Gram-positive bacteria (*Staphylococci, Corynebacteria*), and about 20% of the human population permanently carry *Staphylococci* on the skin. The skin usually resists the resident flora, which survive in the form of colonies with no clinical signs. However, with a decrease in skin resistance they may cause local clinical infection (impetigo, folliculitis, cellulitis, etc.).

Transient flora consist mainly of recent contaminants and can be found only in the superficial layers. They can be removed by cleaning, which can be improved by disinfectants. They are found mainly on the hands or on those skin surfaces that have been in contact with an external source of an infectious agent.

Skin always contains organic substances (proteins, lipids, etc.) that decrease the effect of disinfection, especially fatty skin. This requires cleaning and disinfection in one phase, or precleaning with detergent before disinfection. Fatty and dirty skin needs more detergent, or more frequent repetition and longer exposure, than dry and clean skin.

Different purposes of skin disinfection can be distinguished:

- skin disinfection before invasive procedures:
  - puncture
  - surgical operations
- hand disinfection:
  - hygienic hand disinfection
  - surgical hand disinfection
- whole body disinfection.

Skin disinfection before an invasive procedure is done in order to kill both the resident and transient flora, thus defending the deep and susceptible sterile tissues from the endogenous source of infection. The difference between 'puncture' and 'surgical operation' is the extent of the wound, which is a maximum of 5 mm in a puncture, but can be several centimetres in a wound from a surgical operation. The difference in the size of the wounds determines the number of applications of the disinfectant medium: a puncture will normally require up to three applications, while a surgical operation will need a minimum of five. The larger the wound the greater the number of micro-organisms that can infect the deep tissues, exceeding the infectious dose, hence more micro-organisms have to be killed. The first applications destroy only the transient flora while the subsequent applications will reach the deep layers of the skin, killing the resident flora.

Hand disinfection is one of the most important practices in infection control. It prevents the transmission of an infectious agent via the hands from a source of infection to both the patient and the health care professional.

Ignacz Semmelweis was the first to demonstrate the decrease in mortality from childbed fever (puerperal fever) as a result of hand disinfection with chlorine (Semmelweis, 1861). Figure 5.4 was prepared from Semmelweis's raw data, demonstrating the effect graphically.

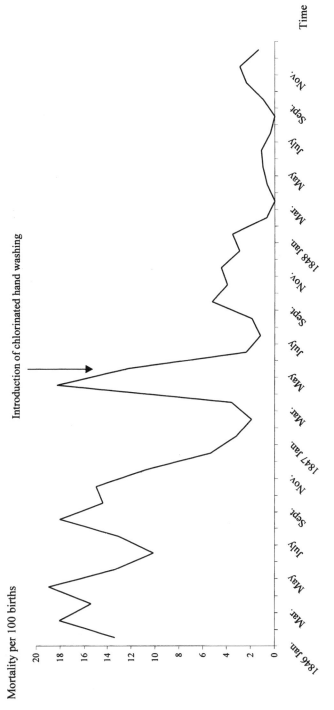

Figure 5.4. Effect of chlorinated hand washing on the mortality of childbed fever at Vienna Maternity Hospital (graph prepared from data of Ignacz Semmelweis, 1861).

Techniques of hand disinfection have greatly improved since the nineteenth century, and these can be classified as:

• immersion
• hand washing
• scrubbing and drying the disinfectant on the skin.

Immersion is done by filling a basin with a solution of chemical disinfectant and immersing the hands for a specified time. This technique was used by Semmelweis, and it was in use until the mid-1960s. Its disadvantage is that the solution must be changed frequently as the concentration of the chemical disinfectant decreases with use and self-depletion over time. The lower concentration does not kill all the micro-organisms, which remain alive in the solution, infecting the hands each time and causing cross-contamination. This method is not recommended for use nowadays.

The hand washing method is applied by using tap water with a detergent-disinfectant, followed by rinsing with tap water. This technique is recommended if the hands are contaminated with lots of organic substance, or are moist. The hand washing technique has several critical aspects:

• The first important point is that if the soap contains only a detergent then the removal of micro-organisms is limited by cleaning, without killing the micro-organisms on the hand. If the soap contains detergent with a chemical disinfectant better disinfection can be achieved by mechanically removing and killing the micro-organisms together.
• The next critical issue is the consistency of the soap (hard soaps or bath soaps, and liquid soaps). Hard soaps cannot be recommended in health care practice, even if they contain chemical disinfectant. They may remain contaminated with micro-organisms after use, because they have been touched by the hand directly, which may lead to cross-transmission of infectious agents. Liquid soaps remove the possibility of cross-transmission, because the soap in the container will not be touched by the hands. Liquid soaps are recommended for use in health care settings.
• The third critical point in the hand washing technique is the risk of recontamination of the hand when it is rinsed with infected tap water (or by contact with the tap).
• Finally, the soap rinsed from the hand has no residual effect on the skin, and thus the effect of the disinfectant is limited to the period of hand washing.

Despite these disadvantages, the hand washing technique remains the most important way to decontaminate hands. It is essential in personal hygiene, both in health care settings and in households.

Scrubbing is the latest method to be introduced for hand disinfection. It does not need water because the disinfectant is left to dry on the skin. Its advantages compared with hand washing methods are that:

- chemical disinfectants using this method have a killing effect, increasing the effectiveness of disinfection compared with soaps containing only detergent
- it is available only in liquid form, so avoiding cross-transmission of infectious agents
- there is no danger of recontamination of the hands by tap water
- disinfectant left on the hands has the residual effect of prolonging the exposure, thus giving more time for the disinfectant to act.

However, scrubbing is less effective than hand washing if the hand is contaminated with substantial amounts of organic substances or moisture which cannot be removed properly by scrubbing.

Both the washing and scrubbing techniques are used for the two main types of hand disinfection: hygienic and surgical.

Hygienic hand disinfection is used for the prevention of transmission of infectious agents from one patient to another during patient care, and for the self-defence of the staff. The aim is to remove and kill the transient flora, which consist mainly of the nosocomial pathogens that have recently contaminated the hands of the staff at work. The hands should be disinfected at any time that they become contaminated by hazardous microorganisms and there is a danger of transmitting them. It is recommended that this be done before and after any type of care for each patient. Any type of washing or scrubbing technique may be used, taking into account the advantages and disadvantages of each method in the particular circumstances.

Surgical hand disinfection is done to prevent the transmission of both resident and transient flora from the hand of the surgeon to the surgical wound if damage to sterile gloves occurs during an operation. The technique is strictly regulated, and the order in which the washing and scrubbing methods are applied cannot be inverted. In the first phase the surgeon or sterile nurse should clean his or her hands with a liquid soap, removing the moisture and organic substances, which of course will remove some micro-organisms as well. In the second phase scrubbing with chemical disinfectants should be done in several applications, which is usually five times for most chemicals. The scrubbing will kill both the residual and transient flora, and the residues remaining on the skin will protect the outer surface from recontamination from the deep tissue layers.

Whole body disinfection is done in order to clean and disinfect the whole body surface if it is dirty or contaminated by an infectious agent that may be a hazard to the host him- or herself or to others in the environment. It is carried out as part of general body hygiene and before scheduled operations.

Skin cannot be sterilized. Skin disinfectants in current use can achieve only selective disinfection. There have been many attempts to find the perfect hand disinfectant. However, a statistically significant decrease in the amount of skin contaminants does not amount to complete disinfection because micro-organisms may survive and be transmitted, but in fewer numbers (Meers et al., 1978). Additionally, handwashing techniques miss areas on the hand because of anatomy and the lack of careful application to all parts of the hand (Taylor 1978a, 1978b). Despite this, hand disinfection cannot be ignored because a reduction in the initial amount of micro-organisms to less than the disease dose (for example in faecal–oral infections) can be achieved only in this way. The use of gloves as a 'removable skin' may compensate for the unavoidable disadvantages of skin disinfectants. Gloves and hand disinfection together are recommended in health care settings.

Hand disinfectants used for scrubbing are usually alcohol based. Alcohols have both cleaning and disinfecting effects. The mixture of different types of alcohol with other substances, for example chlorhexidine, may have a synergistic effect, increasing the anti-microbial spectrum of the disinfectant.

Skin disinfectants remove fatty acids from the skin which have a protective effect, leading to dryness of the hand. Many hand disinfectants contain additives to prevent dryness of the hands. However, it is difficult to develop a disinfectant that cleans the hand and kills all the micro-organisms while keeping the skin fatty and soft at the same time. Hand creams and lotions are recommended for use regularly after shifts or when doing administrative work. Small injuries may be caused by the frequent use of skin disinfectants, which may lead to skin infections from the endogenous resident skin flora, and may serve as a gate for pathogens from an external source, especially blood-borne microbes.

Disinfection of mucosa

Mucosa of organs with an external gate to the environment (respiratory tract, mouth and gut, eye, genital tract) may be colonized by different micro-organisms. Urine is sterile in normal situations. However, mucosa is less resistant to micro-organisms and more vulnerable than intact skin. Disinfection of mucosa is done for several reasons:

- to prevent the invasion of micro-organisms from the surface of the mucosa into the deep tissues during an operation (e.g. orofacial or eye surgery)
- regular disinfection of the urinary tract in patients with a permanent transurethral catheter, to prevent urinary tract infections
- selective decontamination of mouth and throat, preventing nosocomial pneumonia among mechanically ventilated patients
- oral hygiene.

Mucosae can tolerate only those disinfectants that do not have an irritating effect. An alcohol base is not used for this purpose, only water-based disinfectant chemicals (for example chlorhexidine, hexachlorophane, poli/1-vinil-2-pirrolidon/iodine complex, octenidindihidroklorid, etc.) or local antibiotics can be used.

Some disinfectants are licensed for disinfection of both skin and mucosa, but in different concentrations. If the skin-mucosal disinfectant has to be diluted for the disinfection of mucosa, then only sterile water must be used.

Quality control of chemical disinfectants

The aim of quality control of disinfectants is to kill or remove potentially pathogenic micro-organisms in the environment without hazard to those who have direct or indirect contact with the disinfectant agent. Many more chemicals are licensed and produced than are in use in a health care setting at any one time. This requires the appropriate selection of those that fulfil the specific requirements of the given health care setting.

Quality control consists of two practical steps:

- licensing and introduction of disinfectants on the market
- maintenance and everyday use.

The manufacturer is responsible for obtaining a licence and for providing the user with all necessary information about the disinfectant. The hospital infection control committee is responsible for choosing the appropriate disinfectants for local use. The following documents should be provided by the manufacturer when introducing a disinfectant into a health care setting:

- a licence from the national health authority that is in charge of licensing the specific disinfectant, together with a specification of the type of use (skin disinfection, hand disinfection, instrument disinfection, surface disinfection, laundry, etc.)
- the exact contents of the disinfectant (main substances, additives, vehicle, etc.)
- toxicological and safety parameters, appropriate information about all the components of the disinfectant and any possible environmental hazard, and the method of first aid if intoxication occurs
- licensed labelling text and approved instructions for use (concentration, time of exposure, etc.)
- the microbiological spectrum at the specified exposure (i.e. killing effect at the specified concentrations and for different times of exposure).

Chemical disinfectants should be introduced into a health care setting based on cost/benefit and cost/effectiveness principles. Overuse will increase the cost, while keeping effectiveness at the same level; inappropriate use may lead to an increase in HAI. Cost can be taken into account if there are many alternative choices in the same group of disinfectants. Each hospital should have a written 'disinfection policy' containing the list of disinfectants (called the local formula) and their concentrations. The following points should be taken into consideration:

- the known or expected micro-organisms and their resistance to the disinfectant methods
- the anti-microbial spectrum of the disinfectant ('cide' or 'static' effect)
- the characteristics of the item to be disinfected (any damage)
- cleaning and disinfection in one phase or in two phases (cleaning first then disinfection)
- experience of the practical use of the disinfectant
- any residual effect, and its duration
- possible occupational hazard.

Maintenance of the disinfection policy should be controlled in two ways:

- by regular checks on correct use
- by periodic reviews of the disinfection policy.

Disinfectants are used correctly if the manufacturer's instructions are followed (i.e. for the licensed purpose and in approved concentrations). The most critical point is if the disinfectant is incorrectly diluted by the user. The concentration of disinfectants is usually expressed in percentages (%) in SI units (Système International d'Unités). According to this, the dilution in percentage terms means that the solution contains as much of the substance weighed in grams per 100 ml as the percentage of the solution. For example a 1% solution means that one gram of substance is dissolved in 100 cm³ (ml) of the solution. Annexe 3 contains a table showing the appropriate weights of disinfectant to be diluted to achieve the required dilution in percentage terms for different amounts of solution, when 1 cm³ is equivalent to one ml of the solution. If the consistency of the disinfectant is equal to one gram per ml, then the numerical quantity of the disinfectant will be the same in ml as in grams.

It is prohibited to dilute a disinfectant that has already been diluted by the manufacturer, or where the disinfectant is specified for use in concentrated form. Mixtures of different disinfectants are not allowed unless the manufacturer specifically permits it.

Disinfectants should be kept in their original containers or feeders, unless it is allowed to be poured into another feeder for convenience of use or for pumping. The new feeder should, of course, be clearly labelled according to the contents.

A review of disinfection policy is recommended at least annually. There is no need to change the local list unless any of the following circumstances occur:

- the licence is withdrawn by the authority
- the quality of the disinfectants is not consistent owing to poor quality control by the manufacturer
- if an increase in HAI is due to insufficiency of the disinfectant (too narrow a spectrum or the development of resistance), but where inappropriate use can be excluded
- recognition of impracticalities in use
- development of an alternative chemical disinfectant with the same effect but at lower cost

- development and availability of a more effective chemical disinfectant than has been available hitherto.

Antibiotic treatment

Anti-microbial agents (generally known as 'antibiotics') are those agents that are used for killing or inhibiting micro-organisms only within the human or animal body. If the antibiotic treatment leads to the clearance from the host of the infectious agent it helps to interrupt the transmission of the infectious agent. Chemical disinfectants also have an 'anti-microbial' effect, killing or inhibiting micro-organisms, but despite this they are clearly distinguished from antibiotics in medical terminology because of two main differences:

- their anti-microbial spectrum against micro-organisms
- their toxic effect on the host, and the method of application.

The anti-microbial spectrum of a chemical disinfectant is much wider than the antimicrobial spectrum of an antibiotic. A chemical disinfectant acts against a wide range of micro-organisms at the same time, for example against viruses, bacteria, fungi, or even spores, while the action of an antibiotic is limited to only a subgroup of micro-organisms, or even to only one species. This specificity defines the classification of antibiotics into different agents (antiviral, antibacterial, antifungal, antiprotozoal, antiparasitic).

Antibiotics are usually less toxic than chemical disinfectants. Their relatively low toxicity is the reason they can be used in wider applications than chemical disinfectants:

- systematic use internally:
  - parenterally– injections
  - per os – tablets or syrup
- topical use on skin and mucosa.

However, some of the antibiotics can be applied only topically for external use, such as skin-mucosal disinfectants if their toxicity and other pharmacokinetic features allow them for external use only (for example mupirocin).

Antibiotic treatment may be classified into two groups according to the availability of information about the infectious agent and its anti-microbial resistance within an individual host:

- empiric treatment
- target treatment.

Empiric antibiotic treatment is defined as a treatment when the exact infectious agent in an individual case cannot be identified (but may only be suspected), or the antibiotic susceptibility of an identified infectious agent cannot be determined ad hoc, in which case the choice of antibiotic is based on the antibiotic susceptibility results derived from past cases.

Target antibiotic treatment means the infectious agent is known, by culture or by another method derived from the individual host, and the antibiotic susceptibility of the identified infectious agent is determined *in vitro* immediately before treatment, and the treatment is based on this susceptibility pattern.

Antibiotics are used for several treatment purposes with importance in HAI as well. Their main uses can be classified as follows:

- for clinical purposes:
  - therapy of infectious diseases
- for preventive purposes (prophylaxis):
  - at the stage of the susceptible host:
    ○ antibiotic prophylaxis
    ○ selective decontamination (SD)
  - at the stage of the source of the infection:
    ○ decontamination of asymptomatically infected hosts that are a source of a known infectious agent.

Therapy of infectious diseases with anti-microbial agents aims first to cure the clinical disease, preventing death and other complications from the infection. The additional aim of antibiotic therapy can be the clearance from the clinically infected host of the infectious agent, leading to the interruption of the transmission of the infectious agent and being a preventive measure at the same time. However, complete removal cannot be guaranteed and the host may remain the source of an infectious agent even after the disappearance of clinical signs.

As stated previously, antibiotic therapy may be 'empiric' or 'target'. Better results can be expected from target therapy than from empiric therapy because empiric therapy is always a 'guess' as to the infectious agent, or its antibiotic resistance is not known.

The effect of antibiotic therapy is strictly time dependent, i.e. the earlier it is begun the better the chance of a cure without complications. This is important for the further outcomes of any infections, including HAI.

Antibiotic prophylaxis is widely used to prevent both HAI and infections outside hospital. Its aim is to prevent the attachment and growth of an infectious agent in a susceptible host. Generally, antibiotic prophylaxis is empiric as the infectious agent can be only suspected in most cases because its antibiotic resistance is not available. Two types of antibiotic prophylaxis can be distinguished, depending on the temporal relation between the prophylaxis and contact with an infectious agent:

- post-exposure prophylaxis
- pre-exposure prophylaxis.

Post-exposure prophylaxis is when treatment begins after the host has been in contact with a known or suspected infectious agent. An example is when AZT prophylaxis is used after a health care worker is injured by an instrument that has been used for the care of an HIV-infected patient. Another example is the antibiotic given to persons in contact with someone infected with *Neisseria meningitidis*.

Pre-exposure prophylaxis means that the prophylaxis starts before, and it is continued during, the period of contact with a known or suspected infectious agent. An example is the antibiotic prophylaxis used to prevent surgical wound infections during operations. Another example of this type is the chemoprophylaxis used against malaria by travellers to areas where the disease is endemic.

An important condition for all types of antibiotic prophylaxis is that the anti-microbial spectrum of the chosen antibiotic should cover the susceptibility range of the infectious agents against which protection is required.

Antibiotic prophylaxis can be used alone if there is no other method of prevention, or may be added to other preventive measures to increase the efficacy of the prevention. However, it cannot be used alone in the prevention of HAI; it is only a complementary method to the other isolation techniques in hospitals, not a replacement for them.

Selective decontamination (SD) is used to prevent infection from the gut if abdominal surgery involves opening the gut system. It is used against the bacterial flora of the gut, which consist of Gram-negative bacteria of the genera of *Enterobacteriaceae*, Gram-positive *Enterococcus* species, and anaerobic bacteria (mainly *Clostridium* species).

Decontamination of inapparent cases is done purely as a preventive measure to interrupt the transmission of infectious agents into the environment by treating all the hosts who are infected in a relatively small population, or in an outbreak situation. This is done, for example, by prescribing mupirocin for persons colonized with methicillin-resistant *Staphylococcus aureus* (MRSA).

Barriers

Barriers prevent the transmission of an infectious agent in a purely physical way. They are used to prevent the transmission of an infectious agent among humans, or when a person must be protected from some other inanimate vehicle of the infectious agent. In the community the most common barrier technique is the use of condoms to prevent the passage of infectious agents by sexual transmission (HIV, hepatitis B and C, gonorrhoea, syphilis, etc.).

In the health care setting, protection by barriers is achieved by:

* separation of an infected human (infective isolation) or susceptible host (protective isolation)
* wearing barriers.

Separation in a single room of an infected human, as a source of the infection, is also a barrier technique where the walls serve as barriers impeding the spread of the microbes through the air. It is necessary if there is a possibility of direct or indirect transmission of defined infectious agents among roommates within the confines of the room. This applies to respiratory/airborne transmission, and to faecal–oral routes. It is also used for particularly hazardous infections (such as yellow fever, Ebola virus, Marburg virus, Lassa virus, plague, etc). But, for example, hepatitis B carriers do not need a single room unless the patient is a psychiatric case. This type of precaution does not reduce the time during which infectious agents may spread from the source; in this case the level of infectivity may decline only due to the natural processes of the infection. The period of infectivity determines the required period of separation. That is why it is recommended that patients admitted to hospital be separated in a single room for a minimum of 72 hours to identify the imported infection and to assess the further isolation precautions necessary.

Wearing barriers is the second most widely used isolation technique. Here, coats, gloves, goggles, masks, special shoes, and even a 'spacesuit' are used. Non-sterile barriers may harbour an infectious agent, which is a source of infection, so barriers must be sterile if there is a high risk of transmitting an infectious agent to the patient (operating rooms, other invasive procedures, etc.). However, sterility is not required if they are used for protection against an infectious source. However, cross-contamination may occur, and this should be taken into account. Barriers may be contaminated during contact with the direct source, or through the vehicle of the infectious agent, thus they need to be decontaminated because they become the vehicles of further transmission of the infectious agent. Barriers are of great occupational importance for staff to protect themselves against any discharges from patients.

Prevention of transmission of infection at the stage of susceptible host

Prevention of the transmission of an infectious agent at the stage of susceptible host can be done in the following ways (see Figure 5.1, page 117):

- protective isolation (mentioned above)
- barriers (mentioned above)
- antibiotic prophylaxis (mentioned above)
- immunization:
  - for specific immunity:
    - ○ vaccination
    - ○ artificial passive immunization
  - regulation of immune function – immunomodulators.

The aim of immunization is to increase resistance to infectious agents. If the immunization leads to complete resistance to an infectious agent, then it may stop its growth and further spread. The first possible method is intervention at the level of specific immunity by making the host produce specific immune factors or providing him or her with ready-made ones.

Vaccination aims to protect individuals artificially against infectious diseases. The word *vaccination* comes from the name of a virus, 'vaccinia' (causing cowpox), that was used first by the English physician Edward Jenner in 1798. He immunized people with the attenuated virus of cowpox via scarification on the upper arm, recognizing that people working at dairies did not get ill with smallpox if they had previously been ill with cowpox. To date more than 400 microbes have been found to infect humans and about 20 vaccines have been approved against infectious diseases, which may protect against approximately 5% of the total number of infections in humans (Chin, 2000; Mims et al., 2001). 'Vaccinology' as a new sub-science of medicine has been developed in parallel with immunology, which deals with protection generally. Discoveries in immunology have been used in many aspects in vaccinology as they share a common research field.

Infectious diseases against which vaccines have been developed are called 'vaccine-preventable infectious diseases', distinguishing them from other infections. In hospital, the clinical and preventive approach to these infectious diseases is similar to that for infections outside hospital.

As discussed in Chapter 3, both active and passive immunity can be acquired artificially if the specific immunity is acquired by conscious human intervention (vaccination).

In *active artificial immunization,* immunity is achieved only after the self-production of specific immune factors, which takes time; hence it protects the host only after a certain period of time has elapsed from the moment of vaccination. Vaccination can be given orally (such as oral polio vaccine) or by injection into muscle, subcutaneously or intracutaneously, or by scarification into the skin (vaccine against smallpox used to enter in this way).

Vaccination of the human population changes the occurrence and nature of infectious diseases at the population level, which depends on the following determinants (WHO, 1996):

- the mechanism of the direct action of the vaccine
- the vaccine coverage of the population
- characteristics of the infectious agent
- the existence of non-human hosts of the infectious agent.

Direct action of the vaccine confers resistance to an infectious agent in two ways:

- reduction of the severity of the disease – it prevents the more serious consequences of the infection in humans (death, other complications, disability) without influencing the transmission of the infectious agent, because the human is not the principal source of these infections (tetanus, rabies vaccination in humans), or limited inhibition of the transmission of the infectious agent in humans as the principal source of the infection (pertussis)
- resistance to the infection – it prevents serious consequences of the infection and at the same time reduces the transmission of those infectious agents in the human population for which the human population is the only source of infection (measles, poliomyelitis, diphtheria).

Resistance to infection is correlated with the theory of 'herd immunity' – that is the *indirect* action of a vaccine, when a large proportion of the population is vaccinated and this protects even unvaccinated people or those whose immunity has waned (i.e. who are no longer immune) by reducing the transmission (see Chapter 3).

The degree of direct and indirect effects of vaccination can be estimated mathematically by assessing:

- the immunogenicity of the vaccine
- the vaccine efficacy.

Immunogenicity is a characteristic of a vaccine that bestows protection, and is measured by the production of several types and levels of cellular and/or humoral immune factors. It is expressed as the percentage of vaccinated persons reacting to the vaccination by developing those factors. The strength of the immunity is expressed:

- quantitatively (quantity of antibodies, proliferation of immune cells, etc.) after the introduction of a defined amount of antigen
- by the duration of protection.

Immunogenicity is determined by testing on volunteers during the licensing process for the vaccine, or during the post-licence surveillance. Care should be taken to ensure that the volunteers do not acquire their immunity in any way other than through test vaccination (such as exposure to the infectious agent in the community).

The terms 'vaccination' and 'immunization' are not equivalent. If someone is vaccinated it entails only the introduction of a vaccine into the body, but it does not mean that he or she is immunized. A person is immunized if an adequate level of immune factors is produced after the vaccination, which depends entirely on the immunogenity of the vaccine. Immunogenicity of a vaccine is influenced by the characteristics of the vaccinated person reacting to the vaccine (age, gender, immune status, underlying diseases diminishing the immune function, etc.) and by the method of introduction into body.

Vaccine efficacy is expressed as the decrease in the occurrence (incidence) of the disease in the population attributable to the vaccine. The higher the vaccine efficacy the more potential cases are prevented by the vaccine. It is estimated by comparing the frequency of the infectious disease among vaccinated and non-vaccinated individuals. However, the wane of immunity among the population decreases vaccine efficacy over time, even with a high initial immune response but with a short duration of immunity. If the vaccine efficacy is estimated for a pooled population without stratification according to the time of being vaccinated and other determinants, this may erroneously cause the vaccine to be declared ineffective. If the estimated pooled efficacy is low it is advisable to estimate the efficacy for different strata because this can vary with age, gender, geographic area, or it can be different for subtypes of the same infection.

Vaccine coverage is the proportion of the population actually vaccinated against an infectious agent in a certain geographic area. It may rise and fall over time, leaving a proportion of the population unvaccinated if it does not reach 100%. If enough people remain unvaccinated (i.e. non-immune) there may be outbreaks even in those areas where the infectious agent was believed to have been eliminated through the accumulation of susceptible persons (WHO, 1996). The higher the coverage the more prevented cases are to be expected if immunogenicity and efficacy are the same. Vaccine coverage is an important factor to take into account when deciding the minimum proportion of the population to be vaccinated in order to prevent outbreaks and to decrease transmission of the infectious agent with a net reproduction ratio of one (see Chapter 3).

Because all the determinants act at the same time, the expected level of vaccine-preventable HAI may be subject to the following influences:

- a decrease in the prevalence of susceptibility to the specified infection of patients admitted to hospital, staff, and visitors
- a lower probability of being exposed to the infectious agent in hospital, i.e. a decreased prevalence of the infectious agent as a result of localizing that agent to limited sources.

Vaccines used for artificial active immunization can be classified as:

- live-attenuated
- non-viable.

Live-attenuated vaccine contains a standard amount of a viable micro-organism with low virulence. The vaccine strain may complete one or several growth cycles in the host and, depending on the residual virulence of the vaccine, it may cause mild or asymptomatic infection after vaccination. This explains why vaccination with live-attenuated vaccine usually needs fewer doses to achieve the required immunity.

Non-viable vaccine contains a standard amount of killed micro-organism or an extract of those antigens that are responsible for the immunity. Vaccination with a non-viable vaccine usually needs several doses to achieve adequate immunity. This is due to the lack of the growth of the killed strain, or the low immunogenicity of the antigen per single dose to provoke strong immunity (diphtheria, pertussis, tetanus, hepatitis B, tick-borne encephalitis, flu).

Primary vaccination is the first time that someone is vaccinated against an infectious agent. If the vaccinated person has received all the doses required to reach the maximum (adequate) level of immunity achievable with the specified vaccine it is called 'complete vaccination'; if not, it is called 'incomplete vaccination'.

Booster vaccination is when vaccine is given again to a person with previous complete primary vaccination in order to prevent the waning of immunity. For example, for vaccination against hepatitis B (which contains HBsAg) three doses are required for primary vaccination and one booster dose should be given every fifth year after the first dose of complete primary vaccination according to the current recommendation.

Artificial passive immunization is the second main means of making the host immune to an infectious agent (see Chapter 3). However, this process is not true vaccination, and it should be distinguished from vaccination proper to avoid confusion. Preparations that contain ready-made antibodies are called immunoglobulins. The amount of antibody is called the 'titre', which is usually expressed in units per ml (U/ml), or in international units per ml (IU/ml), and it is measured by the inactivation or neutralization of a known amount of microbial antigen. 'Titre' (derived from the word 'titration') involves the serial dilution of antibody, and it describes the highest dilution at which the measured effect is detected. Immunoglobulins may contain antibodies to several micro-organisms or antigens (polyclonal antibodies, PAb), or antibody to only one species or even one subtype (monoclonal antibodies, MAb).

According to the source, both the polyclonal and monoclonal immunoglobulins can be divided into two groups:

*   homologous – made by another human body
*   heterologous – produced by animals (cow, horse, etc.).

Homologous immunoglobulins are prepared from the blood of humans. They are produced by two main methods and in two forms:

*   human gammaglobulin
*   hyper-immune gammaglobulins.

Human gammaglobulin is prepared from plasma of human blood donors. It contains immunoglobulins against infectious agents that were circulating in the blood of donors at the time of donation. According to the content, they are polyclonal. Because the titre of antibodies to different micro-organisms may be different in each person, blood from about one thousand (or more) blood donors is pooled in one batch for balance and to achieve the standard titre of the gammaglobulin produced.

The titre of gammaglobulin against micro-organisms produced in this way reflects the average level of immunity of the population from which the blood donors come. Lack of, or a decrease in, natural active immunization or vaccine coverage or waning of immunity within the general population leads to lack of antibodies, or to their decreased titre in the blood of the general population and hence in donors and in the resulting gammaglobulin. This restricts the use of gammaglobulin produced from blood donors.

The longer the time between infection and the donation of blood, the lower the titre of antibodies to be expected owing to waning of immunity. If donation occurs more than six weeks after infection then only immunoglobulins of class G can be expected in the plasma.

Human hyper-immune gammaglobulins are prepared from the human plasma of 'hyper-immune' people, whose blood contains antibodies to an infectious agent in higher titre than in the general population. This occurs when a person is in the convalescent phase of the natural clinical infection, or the blood is donated a short time after natural inapparent infection or vaccination against an infectious agent.

Human hyper-immune gammaglobolulin not only contains a higher titre of antibodies than gammaglobulin from pooled blood donors, but immunoglobulins of class M and G are to be expected if the blood is taken within six weeks after infection, which is another advantage of hyper-immune gammaglobulin.

Regardless of the type of gammaglobulin, its titre against each type of infectious agent should be checked and reported by the manufacturer.

Heterologous immunoglobulins are prepared from animal plasma after vaccination of the animals (cow, horse, sheep, or other) with an antigen. It is called heterologous because the immunoglobulins come from non-human species. This is an important issue because such immunoglobulins may contain other proteins that behave like an antigen for humans, immunizing the recipient human host by causing allergy. Repeated doses of heterologous immunoglobulin produced from the same animal species can cause serious anaphylactic shock. Allergization may also happen with homologous immunoglobulins, but it occurs less frequently than with heterologous ones.

Vaccination may be grouped according to the target population for whom it is recommended:

- children and adolescents
- inhabitants of areas of high risk, or travellers entering those areas
- high-risk groups.

However, some vaccines can be recommended for more than one target group. For example, the vaccine against hepatitis B is recommended for children, for those in hazardous occupations (health care workers), and also for those with high-risk behaviour – frequent change of sexual partners, bisexuals and homosexuals, being in jail, tattoos (Chin, 2000).

Childhood vaccination consists of the vaccines against infectious agents that contribute to high morbidity and mortality of children, and safe vaccines have been approved for this age group (see Table 5.5). It is noticeable that childhood vaccination consists mainly of those vaccines of infectious agents that are transmitted by the airborne route, falling into the group of respiratory infections that are the most common infections among children. This is explained by the fact that the mucosa of the respiratory tract of children is less resistant to infectious agents.

It is not by chance that it is a requirement of body substance isolation (BSI) that all health care workers should be vaccinated with those vaccines that are recommended for childhood vaccination, and if possible against others transmitted by the airborne route, because it is most difficult to control this group of infections by other isolation techniques (Lynch et al., 1987; Lynch et al. 1990). Health care staff whose airways are infected may very easily transmit the infectious agent throughout the hospital. Additionally, the absence of many health care workers who may be ill at the same time, or for any other reason, may cause a crisis in the care of patients.

Vaccine efficacy against tuberculosis (TB) is not the same in different geographic areas of the world (Rodrigues et al., 1993; Fine, 1989). This explains the difference in the recommendations against TB in childhood in different regions (see Table 5.5). The vaccine 'Bacillus Calmette-Guèrin' (BCG) given in childhood, with acceptable efficacy, may not prevent TB in adults but may prevent meningitis or disseminated TB in children and young adults, which is a reason not to remove BCG from childhood vaccination (Camargos et al., 1988; Rodrigues et al., 1991). These two forms of

Table 5.5 Recommended vaccination for children.

Age at vaccination	World Health Organization (EPI)	United States	United Kingdom	Hungary
Birth	BCG + OPV + HBV*	HBV (up to two months)		BCG (up to six weeks)
1 month		HBV (up to four months)		
1.5 months	D-P-T + OPV + HBV*			
2 months		D-P-T + Hib + OPV	D-P-T (or D-T) + OPV	Hib
2.5 months	D-P-T + OPV			
3 months			D-P-T (or D-T) + OPV	D-P-T + IPV
3.5 months	D-P-T + OPV + HBV*			
4 months		D-P-T + Hib + OPV	D-P-T (or D-T) + OPV	D-P-T + OPV + Hib
5 months				D-P-T + OPV + Hib
6 months		D-P-T + Hib + OPV (up to 18 months) + HBV (up to 18 months)		BCG if no scar on the skin of primary vaccination
9 months	Measles + Yellow fever**			
12 months		Mu-Mo-R + Hib (all up to 15 months) + V + D-P-T (all up to 18 months)	Mu-Mo-R (up to 18 months)	
15 months		D-T-aP (up to 18 months)		Mu-Mo-R + OPV + Hib
3 years				D-P-T + OPV
4 years		D-P-T or D-T-aP + OPV (all up to 6 years) + Mu-Mo-R (up to 6 years or at 11–12 years)	D-T + OPV + (Mo-Mu-R if not given earlier)	
6 years				D-T
10 years			R (girls only if not given previously, up to 14 years) BCG (up to 14 years only for tuberculin-negative children or infancy)	
11 years		D-T (up to 16 years) + HBV (up to 12 years) + V (if not given earlier)		Mu-Mo-R
14 years				HBV1 + HBV2 + HBV3 (schedule: 0-1-6 month) and BCG if tuberculin-negative
15 years		T + OPV (up to 18 years)		

BCG = Bacillus Calmette-Guérin (against tuberculosis), Hib = Haemophilus influenzae B group, D = Diphtheria, P = Pertussis, aP = acellular Pertussis, T = Tetanus, IPV = inactivated poliovirus, OPV = oral poliovirus, Mu = Mumps, Mo = Morbilli, R = Rubella, HBV = Hepatitis B virus, V = Varicella, * where perinatal transmission is frequent, if it is less frequent then the schedule is: one dose at 1.5, at 2.5 and 3.5 months of age, ** in high-risk areas, EPI = Expanded Program on Immunization.

TB are the relevant indicators in the decision whether or not to include BCG in childhood vaccination in a region.

'*Vaccination for international travel*' describes vaccination both for inhabitants in areas of high occurrence and for travellers visiting such areas or countries, because these infections are poorly controlled or have not been eliminated in those areas, thus the risk of such infections is high (WHO, 1996). Such areas are usually in developing countries of the Mediterranean and the tropics. They are are important for HAI in two respects:

- They cause a permanent infection control problem in hospitals in the areas of high occurrence owing to the high probability of their introduction into hospitals.
- Travellers leaving an area of high occurrence can carry the infectious agent with them and on returning home can become ill and hospitalized, thereby importing micro-organisms (dangerous pathogens or rare pathogens) into the hospital as a source of infection.

Vaccinations for travellers to areas of high risk are of two types:

- compulsory vaccinations
- recommended vaccinations.

Compulsory vaccinations for international travel have been subject to International Health Regulation since 1969 and updated by the World Health Organization (WHO). The infections concerned are those of international importance because of the serious consequences if they are transported from the area of occurrence into another by travellers. Vaccination against these diseases must be documented in the '*International Certificate of Vaccination*' issued by the WHO in Geneva, permitting the holder of a valid certificate to enter or leave the controlled area. In 1969 three infections were regulated: cholera (removed in 1973), yellow fever (still valid) and smallpox (removed in 1980).

Recommended vaccinations for international travel are not compulsory but they are advisable for individual protection and to prevent importing infections that have been eliminated or that are very rare in the home countries of travellers. WHO advises travellers to be vaccinated against poliomyelitis, hepatitis A, hepatitis B, diphtheria, tetanus, and typhoid fever. These all have importance in HAI because they can be transmitted within a health care setting.

Travellers returning to their homeland from an area with a high risk of any infection should tell their doctor about their travels during the previous 12 months if they have to consult him/her for any illness. Medical staff should actively ask all admitted patients whether or not they have travelled abroad.

Vaccination for high-risk population is recommended for those who are at increased risk of contacting an infectious agent as a result of their personal circumstances and/or because of the serious consequences of the development of a disease. These may be classified as:

- occupational biohazard
- behavioural risk
- immunocompromised hosts.

An *occupational biohazard* occurs whenever a person may, in the course of his/her work, make contact with any biological substance infected with an infectious agent. It is an important issue in health care because health care workers come into contact directly and indirectly with patients, producing a biohazard for the staff. In addition to childhood vaccination, it is advisable for health care workers to be vaccinated against other infectious agents that occur more frequently in hospitals than in the general population, particularly where the risk of occupational acquisition is high (hepatitis B, hepatitis A). Other professions, such as laboratory workers, dustmen, sewerage or water supply workers, should also be given special consideration. It is advisable for the employer to take responsibility for providing a list of vaccinations required for a specified profession with any biohazard.

Behaviour or lifestyle may be an indication of the need for vaccination associated with high risk, particularly among those who have an increased probability of contacting a source of an infectious agent (frequent change of sexual partners, prostitutes, tattoos, body piercing).

Immunocompromised hosts, who are more susceptible to infectious agents than the general population due to their underlying health condition, are advised to be vaccinated against those infections that may lead to fatal outcome, but without serious complications of vaccination. For example, individuals with functional or anatomical asplenia should be vaccinated against *Haemophilus*, *Pneumococcus* and *Menigococcus*.

Vaccination can also be classified according to the time of infection, as in the case of antibiotic prophylaxis:

* post-exposure
* pre-exposure.

Post-exposure immunization is recommended if there is a risk of developing an infection with a serious outcome and the host is susceptible for any reason at the moment of contact with an infectious agent:

* he/she has not previously been infected naturally
* he/she is unvaccinated
* primary vaccination is incomplete
* there is wane of immunity.

Post-exposure vaccination should be done as early as possible to achieve an adequate level of immunity, usually immediately or within 48 hours of being infected.

Passive post-exposure immunization with available immunoglobulins (gammaglobulin with adequate titre or hyperimmune-gammaglobulin) should be used in the following circumstances:

* if there is no time to achieve immunity by active immunization (the minimal incubation period of the infectious disease is short, less than two weeks)
* for those for whom active immunization is contraindicated regardless of the duration of minimal incubation period for any of the following reasons:
  - pregnancy
  - development of allergy against any component of the vaccine during previous vaccination
  - if the vaccine for active immunization is not available.

Active post-exposure immunization is also appropriate in several circumstances:

* if the incubation period of an infectious disease is quite long (more than two weeks), so that the immunity may develop actively in time to protect the host from disease (rabies);
* for boosting if the host has been immunized against the defined infectious agent but the level of immunity is not adequate at the time of being infected because of the wane of immunity (tetanus, diphtheria);

- against infectious diseases that have a long incubation period and when immunoglobulin is not available, or only at high cost, or the benefit is similar to that from active vaccination.

Active-passive post-exposure immunization is used in rare situations when the immunoglobulins and the antigen are introduced at the same time into the susceptible host (but into different regions). For example, it is recommended to vaccinate against hepatitis B a newborn baby whose mother is a carrier of HBsAg. Another example is if an unvaccinated health care worker is injured during the care of patient who has hepatitis B infection: the health care worker should immediately receive hyperimmune-gamma-globulin against hepatitis B and active vaccination.

Pre-exposure vaccination is recommended if the possible contact with an infectious agent can be estimated in advance, and an adequate level of immunity can be achieved before the time of contact.

Active pre-exposure immunization is recommended if there is enough time for the development of immunity by active means between the vaccination and possible contact with an infectious agent. This type of vaccination is recommended for high-risk groups and for vaccination for international travel.

Passive pre-exposure immunization is recommended only if contact with the infectious agent is certain, but there is not enough time for the active development of immunity because of the urgent need for vaccination. However, this method should be avoided if possible because immunoglobulins administered will circulate for only up to six months, rendering the host susceptible again later. For example, in the past this method was recommended against hepatitis A before the introduction of active vaccine for anyone travelling into an area of high risk.

Immunomodulators are those substances that normalize the host defence mechanisms if the function of the immune system is deficient or hyperactive. The term 'cytokine' is used to describe all modulators of the immune system. It is of Greek origin: *cyto* = cell, + *kinesis* = movement (Churchill's, 1989, p. 427). The cytokines were initially named according to their presumed function (for example, granulocyte colony-stimulating factor), but the newer cytokines are named interleukins and numbered sequentially because most of them have more than one function. Thus in the literature the terms hematopoietic growth factors (GF), interferons (IFN), interleukine (IL) and tumour necrosis factors (TNF) are not different groups of cytokines but simply reflect the history of this nomenclature.

Cytokines produced by a cell (cellular source) regulate the function of another cell (target cell). The cellular source and the target cells of the same cytokine can be different (polycellular) or only one type of cells (monocellular), which makes immunomodulation very complex. The same cytokine may have an antagonistic or synergistic effect depending on the target cell. The overlap and complex pathways of immunologic reaction can be perceived as a '*molecular war*' between the host and the foreign bodies. Our knowledge about cytokines is increasing and more than 20 cytokines have been described to date.

Because of advances in molecular technology, the number of synthesized cytokines and other substances is increasing for clinical use:

- granulocyte macrophage colony stimulating factor (GMCSF);
- granulocyte colony stimulating factor (GCSF);
- interferon alpha (IFN-α);
- interferon gamma (IFN-γ);
- corticosteroids.

The role of cytokines in clinical practice is increasing with the extension of their licence indications. They offer additional hope for the prevention of HAI in immuno-compromised hosts.

Decision-making in isolation policy

It is advised to control all infectious agents that have rational and efficient infection control measures in order to prevent additional deaths or other consequences if they should cause HAI (Chin, 2000). However, decision-making is necessary in order to use the available resources economically. It is important that everyone who is responsible for decision-making in the prevention of HAI should be familiar with the nature of infections, with specific reference to HAI.

Decision-making in isolation policy has several key points:

- whether the infection is transmitted in a direct or indirect way
- whether it is vaccine-preventable or not
- the expected prevalence of susceptible persons admitted to hospital
- the estimated proportion of inapparent and clinical cases of the particular infection
- the consequences of the outcome of clinical infections
- which are the most important pathogens requiring an isolation policy.

It is desirable that each hospital should have an isolation policy. Biohazards will be different according to different infectious agents, and may change over time, so should be followed up.

Alert micro-organisms are those requiring immediate isolation for the following reasons:

- rapid spread through a hospital owing to high transmissibility, and one or both of the following:
  - high lethality, i.e. serious clinical outcome
  - multi-resistance against anti-microbial agents.

The list of alert micro-organisms may change from one region to another. However, the ubiquity of the most common pathogens of HAI results in the same problems occurring worldwide. There follows a non-exhaustive list of alert micro-organisms:

- viruses:
  - Marburg, Ebola, Lassa
- bacteria:
  - Gram-positive:
    - *Streptococcus pyogenes*, especially causing toxic shock syndrome
    - *Staphylococcus* toxic shock syndrome (STSS)
    - methicillin-resistant *Staphylococcus aureus* (**MRSA**)
    - reduced vancomycin-susceptible *Staphylococcus aureus*
    - glycopeptide-resistant Enterococcus strains, e.g. vancomycin-resistant *Enterococcus* (**VRE**)
  - Gram-negative:
    - *Acinetobacter* species, especially *A. baumannii*
    - *Serratia marcescens*
    - Multi-resistant strains of genera *Enterobacteriaceae*, especially extended-spectrum beta lactamase producing (**ESBL**) *Escherichia coli*, and *Klebsiella pneumoniae*
    - *Pseudomonas aeruginosa* strains showing multi-resistance, especially carbapenem-resistant strains
    - *Stenotrophomonas maltophilia*.

The implementation of a hospital isolation policy is largely determined by two factors:

- architectural
- compliance.

The *architectural* aspect or *design* of the hospital is an essential precursor in the implementation of an effective isolation system. This means that the hospital buildings must satisfy all the architectural requirements that provide appropriate circumstances for the implementation of an isolation policy if it is needed during the functioning of the hospital. If the design of the hospital is not congruent with the principles of isolation, it cannot be compensated for or corrected later! Although it is not the aim of this book to provide details of architectural requirements, it is essential that health care professionals should be familiar with the important aspects. The main architectural elements of an isolation policy may be grouped as follows:

- an adequate number of single rooms
- effective ventilation
- promotion of hand washing
- appropriate degree of cleanliness for storage and transport of equipment.

An *adequate number of single rooms* is crucial and is normally expressed as the proportion of single rooms compared with the total number of beds in the hospital. Single rooms are needed to separate patients for different reasons:

- epidemiological – people with infections transmitted directly, and also those who can transmit the infectious agent to roommates indirectly within the room (such as via the toilet, etc.)
- according to the severity of the illness
- the right of a patient to privacy and individual rest.

These factors require that a certain proportion of beds should be in single rooms in any event. On average 7–10% of patients admitted to hospital acquire HAI and may need separation for some reason, but this figure may rise to 50% or more in high-risk departments (intensive care units, etc.). The perfect solution would be if all the beds in a hospital were in single rooms, but this is affordable only in rich countries, or in private hospitals, owing to high cost. If the number of single rooms is about 30% or more, ideal circumstances exist to deal with separation of patients who need this for any reason. It is no longer recommended that hospitals are built with more than three beds per room. It is also recommended that a sluice room be attached to every patient room, where staff can change their coats and gloves and wash their hands so as not to carry infectious agents from room to room.

Good ventilation is important for controlling airborne infections in both infective and protective isolation cases. Appropriate air pressure gradients prevent the transmission of air droplets and dust from the source of the infection to other areas.

Promotion of hand washing must be achieved at the design stage of the architecture, by specifying an adequate number of sinks for hand washing at every point where it is essential:

- in each patient's room and in the sluice room
- in rooms where any diagnostic or therapeutic procedures (both invasive and non-invasive) are carried out.

The *degree of cleanliness* in the design of hospitals means the total separation of the storage and transport of sterile, clean equipment from any waste throughout the hospital. Its aim is to prevent the contamination of clean and sterile equipment by waste. Separation of the hand washing area from the area for disinfection of equipment falls into this category; disinfection activities always produce aerosols, which may lead to the undesirable spread of infectious agents.

Compliance means the acceptance and appropriate use of the available resources by the management and staff in implementing an isolation policy. It is an ethical issue that every HAI should be prevented if possible, given the local circumstances. The hospital bed, like a coin, has two sides: the patient and the staff. Health care workers should remember that HAI is indiscriminate, and that they too may become patients!

Summary

In summary, the following important points should be highlighted:

- Isolation of infection is *not* equivalent to separation or isolation of the source of the infectious agent, because other isolation techniques are also used to prevent the transmission of infectious agents at other stages.
- Vaccination, by preventing infections, also contributes to the isolation of infections but in a specific way, while for other types of infection non-specific preventive techniques are used because they are applied in all cases, so only the difference in the transmission should be taken into account.
- Non-specific isolation techniques fall into two broad categories (decontamination by sterilization or selective disinfection) and barriers (single rooms and apparel).

- Procedure-independent HAI needs the same isolation techniques as infections outside hospital (Chin, 2000).
- Procedure-dependent HAI requires a special approach but the general issues of isolation techniques should also be used, emphasizing both the external and the endogenous source of the infectious agent and the important fact that the endogenous source of the infectious agent is always present.
- The same isolation technique (for example decontamination) can be used at different stages of the transmission of infectious agents, thus their aim and specifications should be taken into account in any given problem.

Finally, here is a general checklist of when to use similar and different isolation techniques at the three stages of transmission of an infectious agent:

- external animate source of infection:
  - at the stage of the source of the infectious agent:
    - barrier – separation in a single room (infective)
    - ratio of nurses to patients is one to one
    - decontamination of the source:
      - disinfection of the skin (whole body)
      - antibiotics (local or systemic)
  - at the stage of the mode of the transmission:
    - use of disposable equipment – treat it as infectious waste
    - use of barriers (coat, mask, gloves) and their decontamination as possible vehicles for further spread (see below)
    - decontamination of all the vehicles of the infectious agent existing at the time:
      - complete disinfection (sterilization)
      - selective disinfection
      - incineration of infectious waste
  - at the stage of susceptible host:
    - barrier – separation of the susceptible host in a single room (protective)
    - increase of the resistance of the host by specific methods:
      - vaccination for active immunization
      - immunoglobulins for passive immunization
      - immunomodulators
    - antibiotic prophylaxis (local or systematic)

- endogenous source of infection (always present!) in the case of invasive procedures:
  - decontamination before the invasive procedure:
    - selective disinfection of skin and mucosa
    - antibiotic prophylaxis (local or systemic)
    - selective decontamination of the gut.

CHAPTER 6

Common hospital-acquired infections in developed countries

Urinary tract infection (UTI)

Urinary tract infection is one of the most frequently detected hospital-acquired infections (HAI) in health care (Thoburn et al., 1968). However, their occurrence as community-acquired infections (CAI) is also common (Stamm et al., 1989; Stamm and Hooton, 1993). The term 'urinary tract infection' encompasses the infection of different anatomical localizations of the urinary tract: urethritis, cystitis, pyelitis and pyelonephritis.

Aetiology of urinary tract infections

In the aetiology of urinary tract infections the Gram-negative bacteria (*Pseudomonas spp.*, and *Acinetobacter spp.* and members of the *Enterobacteriaceae*: *Escherichia coli*, *Klebsiella spp.*, *Proteus spp.*, *Serratia spp.*), fungi (mainly *Candida spp.*) and *Chlamydiae* play a role, but the distribution of these infectious agents in hospitals is shifted to Gram-negative bacteria, and the role of *Chlamydiae* is much greater in community than in hospital acquisition. In community acquisitions, other microbes like gonococcus are also of importance, but are not common in HAI.

However, *Chlamydiae* need different diagnostic techniques from other microbes. Routinely microbiological laboratories test the urine for *Chlamydiae*, unless there is a special request to do otherwise. If they can be detected, then it is more likely that the infectious agent has been imported to the hospital.

Definition and diagnostic approach of urinary tract infections

Urinary tract infection is a process when a microbe attaches and grows in the urinary tract systems causing inflammation or no host reaction (inapparent UTI).

Diagnosis of UTI is based on detection of the inflammation process and/or the presence of a microbe in the urinary tract using:

- laboratory methods
- image methods.

Laboratory methods serve to confirm the presence of inflammation by pyuria (ten or more white blood cells in one microscopic field or in 1 μl of urine). Microbiological methods use identification methods (see Chapter 1) to demonstrate the presence of a micro-organism.

Image methods (X-ray, isotope, ultrasonography, endoscopy) may confirm the infection if it causes an inflammation.

Microbiological diagnosis of UTI can be:

- qualitative
- quantitative.

Qualitative microbiological identification relies only on the presence of a microbe without determination of its quantity per unit of urine. It is used for *Chlamydia* or *Neisseria gonorrhoeae* or fungi. Smear or other detection methods (PCR) are used for identification of such microbes (see Chapter 1).

Quantitative microbiological identification has been accepted for most Gram-negative and Gram-positive bacteria in order to define a limit of significance – colony-forming unit (CFU) per ml of urine – with the assumption that if the amount of microbe is lower than the limit the UTI is questionable. It is defined by the culture method. However, the quantity of microbe found in the urine at the laboratory depends on the initial amount of the micro-organism in the urine at the moment of collection, and the time between collection and the beginning of laboratory testing. If the test begins more than one hour after collection, then the final amount will be significantly higher due to the growth of the microbe in the urine, which leads to a false high count.

By convention, a bacterial count of $\geq 10^5$ CFU/ml has been accepted as of significance. However, the presence of microbes lower than this limit also confirms infection if contamination of the urine can be excluded (Stark and Maki, 1984). It was confirmed that low-level bacteriuria (10^2 CFU/ml or less) may be accepted as a significant level in women or children, or it may progress rapidly to 10^5 CFU/ml or higher in catheterized patients (Stark and Maki, 1984). Single urine culture gives only a snapshot result because fast-growing bacteria may achieve the 10^9 CFU/ml level in the urine within 72 hours, thus a low bacterial level indicates the early phase of UTI.

In clinical practice, it is advisable to carry out at least two or three urine analyses, especially from urine collected by the midstream method, on consecutive days to exclude the possibility of contamination and to estimate the microbial count in the urine. If consecutive results give the same isolate independently from the bacterial count then the result can be accepted as valid, thus confirming UTI. Inapparent UTI happens more often in patients with transurethral catheters, and the appearance of pyuria confirms clinical UTI, even though there is an absence of subjective complaints.

Classification of urinary tract infections

Urinary tract infections can be classified in several ways, that are important for both clinical and infection control:

- *Anatomical localization of UTI* can be on the lower (urethritis, cystitis, prostatitis) or upper (pyelitis, pyelonephritis) urinary tract.
- *The outcome of UTI* can be clinical infection (pain in the urinary tract, increased frequency and/or urgency of urination, fever and pyuria or microbes in the urine) or inapparent (bacteriuria without clinical signs or pyuria if its other causes – polycystic kidney, analgetic nephrotic syndrome – can be excluded).
- *The frequency of the UTI* can be acutely sporadic (first occurrence), recurrent (two acute episodes within six months or three or more within two years) caused by different microbes, or relapsing (same frequency as recurrent but caused by the same microbe).
- *Predisposing factors* play a role in the increased risk of developing UTIs, and they are classified into two main groups:
  - uncomplicated (no functional or anatomical obstruction, or no invasive procedure on urinary tract)
  - complicated (functional or anatomical obstruction of the urine flow, the insertion of a device into the urinary tract, or surgery, or other factors such as diabetes mellitus, etc.).

Pathogenesis of urinary tract infection

The urinary tract, as a cavity organ, has direct contact with the environment through the urethra. Normally urine contains no microbes. However, the end of the urethra is always colonized (see Chapter 1) but the upper part of the urinary tract is protected by the local defence mechanism (continuous flow of urine, epithelium and sphincter muscles) or by the acidity of the urine, which may also play a defensive role.

UTI may develop by two mechanisms:

- haematogenous spread
- ascending infection.

Haematogenous spread occurs if the urinary tract becomes infected by an infectious agent from another part of the body via sepsis. The appearance of *Staphylococcus aureus* in the urine happens via passive filtration through the glomerula in the kidney, which is the result of secondary spreading from primary foci of the infection.

Ascending spread (transurethral) of UTI occurs when the infectious agent originates from an external source, spreading from the urethral system towards the kidneys. As previously stated, the *predisposing factors* are complementary essential causes of the development of UTI.

In *uncomplicated transurethral* UTIs, no predisposing factors can be found. Haemorrhagic cystitis of sexually active women caused by *Escherichia coli* is the most important CAI, which is explained by the increased adherence of this microbe to the epithelium of the urinary tract. A further form is the urethritis caused by *Neisseria gonorrhoeae* or *Chlamydia*, which is also common in CAIs. Uncomplicated UTI is not common as an HAI, and occurs in very rare situations.

Complicated transurethral UTI occurs if there is a predisposing factor that increases the risk of the development of urinary tract infection. It occurs in both the community and in hospitals, but is much more frequent than uncomplicated UTI as an HAI. According to the predisposing factors, such infections can be classified as:

- retention:
  - anatomical obstruction
  - functional obstruction
- diabetes mellitus (sugar in the urine)
- kidney stones
- increased acidity of the urine toward basic pH
- switch-off of the sphincter function and epithelial defence:
  - reflux of the urine
  - procedure-associated:

  - ○ transurethral catheter
  - ○ endoscopy
- suprapubic urine catheter.

Diabetes mellitus contributes to the development of UTI by the appearance of sugar in the urine, which becomes an excellent medium for the growth of microbes.

In *disturbed acid-base balance* the pH of urine may increase towards basic, which also promotes the growth of microbes.

Retention due to an anatomical anomaly is the main predisposing factor of disturbed urine flow in children (especially in boys) while a functional cause (disturbed nerve regulation of urination) may affect both children and adults. A continuous flow of the urine out of the urinary tract may prevent the urinary tract from being infected; however, if it is disturbed, the micro-organism may remain and grow in the urinary tract, especially in the urinary bladder.

Kidney stones are a risk factor for UTI in adults and they are the most common predisposing risk factor for recurrent complicated urinary tract infection in the community.

Switching off the sphincters and epithelial defence leads to a decrease in the local defence mechanism. It is the most common factor in the development of complicated UTI, and it is the most frequent and essential factor of HAI.

Reflux is the regurgitation of the urine back from the urethra into the urinary bladder, which occurs during urination as a result of inappropriate sphincter function. It occurs mainly in young boys.

Procedure-associated UTI develops due to a decreased local defence of the urinary tract. It is the most common HAI, and is influenced by two factors:

- the extremely high risk of development of UTI due to invasive urinary tract procedures
- the high frequency of urinary tract procedures in hospitals, especially among adults.

The increased risk of development of UTI among catheterized patients is illustrated in Table 6.1 by the different distribution of UTI among patients with and without internal urinary tract catheter.

Procedure-associated transurethral UTI may develop in an *intraluminal* way (inside the indwelling instrument) or *extraluminal* way (between the external surface of the indwelling device and host tissues – the epithelium

Table 6.1. Distribution of urinary tract infections among 341 inpatients on two limb surgery wards at hospital 'A', Hungary, between 2 January and 31 March 1995

	Urinary tract infection		Total
	Yes	No	
Transurethral catheter	18	47	65
No urinary catheter	3	273	276
Total	21	320	341

Cumulative incidence (CI) among catheterized patients: 27.69 UTI/100 catheterized patients, CI among non-catheterized patients: 0.10 UTI/100 non-catherized patients, relative risk: 25.48 (95% confidence interval: 7.73–83.91), Fischer's exact test: $p < 0.0000001$.

of the urethra). The common mechanism of the intraluminal and extraluminal development of UTI during any invasive procedure is injury of the epithelium, through an increased attachment of microbes to the epithelial surface of the urinary tract (Daifuku and Stamm, 1986). Blood during the invasive procedure confirms the injury, but small injuries may not cause bleeding. Blood also serves as a nutritional substance for micro-organisms.

A further effect of invasive procedures – especially in chronically catheterized patients – is the permanent switching off of the sphincters, thus opening the gates for invasion of micro-organisms from the urine collector up to the urinary tract. Particularly successful invaders are Gram-negative bacteria that not only attach to the epithelium of the urinary tract, but also have a natural invasive feature due to the cell structure (fimbria, pili) being able to move even against gravitational force from the collector lower down the urinary tract.

Transurethral catheterization occurs if the catheter is placed in the urinary tract via the urethra. It can be short or long term and it is carried for two reasons:

- medical indication
- for ease of patient care.

The medical indications for inserting a transurethral catheter should be limited to the following reasons:

- retention of urine:
  - anatomical obstruction in the urine flow

– functional obstruction
• daily urine volume measured in a non-cooperating patient.

Anatomical obstruction occurs if there is damage to the structure of the urinary tract, which leads to the retention of urine, and only an internal catheter can maintain the flow. This is the case in trauma or neoplasm, which can be permanent or temporary.

Functional obstruction of the urine flow is due to a disturbance to the neurological regulation of the urine flow, which is important for the contraction of the urinary bladder with the opening of the sphincter at the same time. Several neurological diseases lead to disturbed urination, which can also be temporary (e.g. spinal anaesthesia, deep narcosis during an operation) or permanent (sclerosis multiplex, etc.).

Daily urine volume measure can be the third medical indication in patients who are non-cooperational (or unconscious), when it is extremely important to estimate the daily water and mineral balance with appropriate control of the kidney function (creatinine clearance), or in diabetes to measure the sugar balance. If the patient is conscious enough to co-operate, transurethral catheterization should be avoided.

Ease of patient care is *not* a medical indication to put a transurethral catheter into the patient. It is a convenience for nurses in their care of the patient. It should be avoided, as it is unnecessary and leads to UTI.

The *suprapubic urinary catheter*, which is inserted via the abdominal wall, has been developed to promote the flow of the urine when a transurethral catheter cannot achieve it. This is the case in severe trauma or neoplastic diseases affecting the urethra. A suprapubic urinary catheter does not decrease the occurrence of UTI and, being an invasive procedure of the urinary tract, may cause additional complications (fistula, intra-abdominal infections). It should be used only under rigorous medical direction where the transurethral catheter is contraindicated.

Endoscopy of the urinary tract is an important diagnostic and therapeutic short-term procedure in patients with urological disorders. The development of transurethral operations – such as transurethral resection (TUR) of the prostate – has increased the frequency of endoscopic procedures, thus increasing the number of patients at risk of developing UTI.

Both short- and long-term procedure-associated UTIs may occur during the insertion of the device or during a maintenance operation, which may last minutes (cystoscopy) or be lifelong (chronic transurethral catheterization).

For long-term procedures, the principle is that the closer the infection is to the insertion, the more likely it is to be due to lack of asepsis; and the longer the time between the insertion and the infection, the more likely it is that the infection originated during the maintenance period.

Prevention of urinary tract infections

Urinary tract infection can be minimized, but it cannot be eliminated entirely owing to the presence of predisposing factors and medical indication for invasive urinary tract procedures (Stamm, 1975).

First, it is important to limit the use of invasive urinary tract procedures to those patients with a strong medical indication, and use other methods to assist 'ease-patient care', such as:

- an external 'condom-catheter' for men with incontinence
- disposable nappies.

A preventive strategy for both short- and long-term invasive procedures will entail several different elements:

- aseptic insertion of the device
- aseptic maintenance of the device
- an increase in the local defence mechanism
- a reduction in the amount of micro-organisms to below the disease dose (see Chapter 2).

Aseptic insertion of the device prevents the attachment of microbes from both external and endogenous sources (such as the outer surface of the urethra). Necessary precautions are:

- sterile instruments must be used for catheterization (catheter, bag, etc.)
- the avoidance of contamination of the instruments during insertion:
  - hand disinfection and sterile gloves for staff during insertion
  - sterile linen
- disinfection of the urethral entrance.

Aseptic maintenance of the device prevents late UTI by avoiding microbial contamination of the drainage system by using the following techniques:

- closed drainage:

- two-deck bag system
- closed one-deck bag system
- emptying of the bag in sterile circumstances
- collecting urine by the aspiration method for laboratory testing using sterile syringes and needles without opening the closed system.

An increase in the local defence mechanism aims to provide inappropriate conditions for the presenting microbe to attach and to cause infection:

- injection of sterile anti-microbial gel before the insertion, which prevents damage to the epithelium of the urinary tract
- increase of the acidity of the urine (e.g. mandelic acid).

A reduction in the amount of micro-organism to below the disease dose aims to prevent clinical UTI, especially in chronic catheterized patients, because the micro-organisms may adhere to the surface of the catheter and become a permanent source, thus maintaining the UTI (Nickel et al., 1985). This may be achieved by:

- regular (weekly) changes of the catheter in long-term catheterization
- washing the urinary bladder with mucosal disinfectant (octenidine or poli/1-vinil-2-pirrolidon/iodine complex) every 7–10 days.

Parenteral or oral antibiotics cannot prevent procedure-associated UTI; they should be reserved for the treatment of clinical UTI or for any residual UTI after the removal of the device.

Wound infections

Wound infections arise among patients undergoing surgery, and are the second most frequent HAI, which may reach 30% of all surgical procedures (Thoburn et al., 1968).

Definition and mechanism of wound development

A wound (*vulnus*) is defined as a break in the integrity of any tissue (mucosa, skin, connecting tissue, muscle, etc.) or any organ due to physical (contusion, sharp instrument) or chemical (burn) agents. Different wounds have been defined, and their classification according to the mechanism of their development is important because it characterizes the type of wound and the amount of tissue necrosis, which affect the wound healing process or the development of inflammation. Thus wounds can be classified as: incised wound (*vulnus incisivum*), bite (*vulnus morsum*), jagged or lacerated wound (*vulnus scissum*), bruise (*abrasio*), stab or puncture wound (*vulnus punctum*), contused wound (*vulnus contusum*).

Sources of infectious agents and the aetiology of wound infection

Infectious agents in wound infections may originate from the endogenous skin or mucosal flora where the wound occurs (see Chapter 1), or from exogenous sources from the time of wounding until the wound is healed.

The cause of wound infection depends on the type, the localization and the circumstances of wounding, and especially the agent (knife, scalpel, scissors, bullet, etc.) that causes the wound harbouring the infective agents. In 60% of all surgical procedures, *Staphylococcus aureus*, which inhabits all parts of the skin, is the primary cause of hospital-acquired wound infection. It may come from an endogenous (patient's own flora) or exogenous source (skin flora of the staff) (Bethune et al., 1965; Rammelkamp et al., 1964). The role of coagulase-negative *Staphylococci* of the skin increases in non-human implants (for example, hip replacement). The remaining wound infections are caused by Gram-negative bacteria (*Enterobacteriaceae*, *Pseudomonas*, *Acinetobacter spp.*) and anaerobic microbes. Gram-negative bacteria play a role in the super-infection of primary wound infections caused by *Staphylococci*, but they can also cause primary wound infection, for example *Pseudomonas* in a gunshot wound. Anaerobic bacteria (*Clostridia*, *Peptostreptococcus*, *Bacteroides*) are important in abdominal surgery and traumatic wounds.

Definition and pathogenesis of wound infection

Wound healing problems occur if the edge of the wound does not start to scar by first intention; this is called *dehiscence*. It has a Latin origin: *dehiscentia*; from *dehiscere* = to split open, to develop a gap (Churchill's, 1989, p. 489). Dehiscence can be due to inflammation caused by a micro-organism or have a non-infectious origin as the result of a lack of biological reaction by the host to the wound. There is a risk of developing inflammation of the wounding until it is completely healed.

The definition of wound infection has been a much disputed question among surgeons. Many claim that a wound is infected only if pus appears in it. However, purulent discharge is only one pathological form of wound inflammation (other types are serous, fibrinous fluids) and the classical triad of inflammation – pain (*dolour*), redness (*colour*), oedema (*tumour*) – are also signs of clinical wound infection. Inflammation in general is defined as the tissue and systemic reaction of the organism to any foreign body (e.g. a micro-organism) with increased permeability of the blood vessels, exudation of plasma, and migration of different white blood cells as a result of chemotaxis.

Endogenous bacterial flora is always present, therefore every wound is infected but not every wound will show inflammation, depending on the micro-organism–host reaction (see Chapter 2). Thus, wound infections follow the same classification rules for the outcome of infectious processes as other infections:

- inapparent wound infection
- wound inflammation.

Therefore, definitions of wound infections that rely solely on clinical signs are inappropriate. The term 'wound infection' has a wider meaning, which is not just restricted to inflammation. Admittedly, in practice, inapparent wound infection is not of great importance, as it usually heals without complication. However, with the ever-presence of microbes in even in a completely healed wound, it is important to understand why not every wound is inflamed.

The inflammation process may involve the superficial part of the wound (skin and subcutaneous tissue) and/or the deep soft tissues (fascia and muscles) with or without the involvement of organs or spaces. It is an important fact that deep inflammation may occur without superficial inflammation (the primary healing process of the skin and subcutaneous tissues), showing different clinical signs, but this should be recognized as deep wound inflammation.

In 1992 the Centers for Disease Control (CDC), Atlanta, changed earlier definitions to provide clarification of 'deep infection', omitting the word 'wound' and replacing it with the term 'incisional site', with the explanation that CDC now restricts the term 'wound' to the skin and to the deep soft tissues caused by incision (Garner et al., 1988; Horan et al., 1992a, 1992b).

Careful application is needed if the CDC definition is chosen, because it defines only the *incisional* type of surgical intervention, omitting the other mechanisms of wound development. For example, puncture is another main wounding mechanism for many surgical interventions (e.g. diagnostic puncture of ascites). Furthermore, the CDC definition excludes the other infectious wound complications such as stitch abscess (at the points of suture penetration). It is surprising that the CDC does not recognize episiotomies and circumcision as operative procedures (Horan et al., 1992a, 1992b).

A critical point in the CDC definition is the 'window period' between the wounding and the first clinical sign. CDC has recommended 30 days for superficial and deep incision sites, while for non-human implants it is one year. Deep tissue infections, without superficial wound infections, may develop because of haematogenous spread from distant tissues that have no connection at all with the wound. Implants behave as *locus minoris resitentiae* where bacteria may attach during bacteraemia even after the wound has healed. Thus, the one-year limit for non-human implants should be viewed critically.

The concept of *disease dose* has been applied to explain the development of wound inflammation, using a quantitative measure of microbes in the wound by estimating the minimal microbial count required to cause the inflammation process (see Chapter 2; Foster and Hutt, 1960; Raahave et al., 1986; Mims et al, 2001). In the case of *Staphylococcus aureus*, it was found that the degree of wound inflammation depends on the initial inoculums in the wound and not on the different sources of the strains with assumed differences in virulence. However, this last has not been investigated completely (Foster and Hutt, 1960). A dose of 10^6 CFU/cm^2 of wound has been found to be the disease dose, while if it was less than 10^2 CFU/cm^2 no inflammation occurred, thus confirming that all wounds are infected but the inflammation process is dose dependent (Raahave et al., 1986).

A *microbiological classification* of a wound has been introduced by the National Research Council (NRC) in the USA, which takes into account the site of the operation and other factors (e.g. lapse in technique) that may influence the microbial count (see Table 6.2) (Howard et al., 1964).

In practice, this system helps to compare different types of operations, grouping them according to the likelihood and the degree of microbial contamination at the time of the operation, or until wound closure if no exact microbial count is available (Howard et al., 1964; Cruse and Foord, 1980; Haley et al., 1985a, 1985b; Olson and Lee, 1990; Culver et al., 1991).

As previous stated, every wound should be considered to be contaminated. According to this, the NRC's terminology seems incorrect. A 'clean wound' is also contaminated, but the difference among classes lies in the

Table 6.2. Microbiological classification of wounds and expected wound inflammation

Original NRC-classes[1]	Alternative name of classes	Characteristics of the wound[1]	Expected wound infection per 100 wounds				
			Year of observation				
			1960–62	1967–77	1975–76	1977–86	1987–90
			Year of publication				
			Howard et al., 1964	Cruse and Foord, 1980	Haley et al., 1985b	Olson and Lee, 1990	Culver et al., 1991
					range according to **SENIC** risk index (all)		range according to **NNIS** risk index (all)
Refined-clean*	A	Elective operations, not drained, primary closed	ND	ND	ND	ND	ND
Other clean*	B	No inflammation, no lapse in technique, no entry into gastrointestinal, respiratory except of incidental appendectomy or transection of the cystic duct in the absence of inflammation. Entrance into the genitourinary or biliary tract if the urine or the bile were sterile	5.1	1.5	1.1–15.8 (2.9)	1.4	1.0–5.4 (2.1)
Clean-contaminated	C	Operation on gastrointestinal or respiratory tract with significant spill. Minor lapse in technique, entry into urinary and biliary tract if the urine or bile is infected	10.8	7.7	0.6–17.7 (3.9)	2.8	2.1–9.5 (3.3)
Contaminated	D	Major lapse in technique, acute bacterial inflammation without pus, spillage from gastrointestinal tract, or fresh traumatic wound from relatively clean source	16.3	15.2	4.5–23.9 (8.5)	8.4	3.4–13.2 (6.4)
Dirty	E	Presence of pus, perforated viscus, old traumatic wound or from dirty source	28.0	40.0	6.7–27.4 (12.6)	ND	3.1–12.8 (7.1)

[1] = after Howard et al.; * = in practice later combined into one category 'clean'; NRC = National Research Council; ND = not determined; SENIC = Study of the Efficacy of Nosocomial Infection Control; NNIS = National Nosocomial Infection System.

degree of microbial count per unit of wound. That is why the original category names have been replaced with the alphabetical letters A, B, C, D and E expressing the increase of the possible microbial count in the wound. This modification of terminology avoids confusion and correlates with the wound microbiology and disease dose. This classification has also been used to predict the probability of wound inflammation.

Risk factors of wound infections

There has been much research to discover both the endogenous and exogenous risk factors of wound infections, which together influence the outcome of wound contamination. This is based on the recognition that a reduction of the microbial count in the wound to zero is not achievable, which is confirmed by the continual occurrence of wound infections in wound classes 'A' and 'B' even with improved aseptic preventive techniques. Furthermore, appropriate comparison of the frequency of wound infection is needed as a factor in risk control.

The Study of Efficacy of Nosocomial Infection Control (SENIC), initiated by the Centers for Disease Control (CDC) in 1974, found four risk factors with roughly equal weight adding a score of 1 for each of them that is present (Haley et al., 1985a, 1985b):

- abdominal operation
- operation lasting more than two hours
- contaminated or dirty wound class according to the NRC system
- three or more discharge diagnoses for one patient.

The combination of these four risk factors contributed to five risk-index groups (0, 1, 2, 3, 4) (Haley et al., 1985a, 1985b). Interestingly, the risk of wound infection achieved 15.8/100 operations in the clean wound class in the highest risk-index group (risk index = 3 for this group) (see Table 6.2) (Haley et al., 1985a, 1985b). The ratio of the lowest to the highest infection risk was: in the clean wound class 14.4; in the clean-contaminated 29.5; while in the contaminated and in the dirty it was only 5.3 and 4.1, respectively. This suggests that the above-mentioned risk factors had a greater influence in the development of wound infection in the clean and clean-contaminated groups than in the contaminated or dirty groups.

The CDC later developed a modified version of the SENIC risk indexes in the National Nosocomial Infection System (NNIS) (Culver et al., 1991).

This system allowed only three risk factors to be taken into account:

- the wound class remained in the risk index;
- the ASA (American Society of Anesthesiologists) score (3, 4, 5) was used instead of the number of discharge diagnoses (see Chapter 4);
- a one-point score was assigned if the duration of the operation was above the 75th percentile characteristic of the given procedure, instead of the two-hour limit.

Thus, the NNIS risk index had a score of 0 to 3 because the risk factor for abdominal surgery was eliminated. The risk factors of the NNIS index had a smaller influence on the stratified risk of wound infections than in the SENIC study because the ratio of the lowest to the highest risk was: in the clean class 5.4, in the clean-contaminated 4.5, in the contaminated 3.9 and in the dirty 4.1. However, the NNIS study, conducted about ten years later, showed that the range of the risk of wound infection was also narrower than in the SENIC study, which may reflect the improvement of preventive efforts or a change in the detection system (see Table 6.2; and Chapter 7).

As stated in Chapter 4, the ASA score is quite unreliable because of subjective decision-making, which may lead to misclassification of cases according to the final risk index.

Both the SENIC and NNIS risk indexes may serve for a rough comparison of wound infections, but be of little use to discover and influence other risk factors.

Endogenous risk factors of wound infections are mainly non-specific, i.e. can be found in other forms of HAI. Among them age, diabetes, obesity and hypoalbuminaemia have been found to indicate increased risk of wound infection, and this may be explained by decreased host defence. The co-operation of the patient is important, especially in the post-operative period.

Exogenous risk factors are mainly associated with several phases of the operation (see below), and they may increase the microbial count in the wound or increase local susceptibility in relatively low disease doses:

- preoperative preparation of the patient and operative site
- intraoperative events
- postoperative wound care.

Preoperative preparation of the patient and the operative site aims to decrease the microbial count at the moment of wounding. The lack of whole body disinfection (see Chapter 5) is controversial, while hair removal by clipping or shaving, especially several hours before the operation, had a higher risk than using a depilatory (Seropian and Reynolds, 1971). This is explained by the tiny cuts and subsequent increased growth of local flora. The most critical point is the lack of skin disinfection or its rough-and-ready application at the site of the operation. The presence of 'windows' (where no contact occurs with the disinfectant – see Chapters 3 and 5) on the skin leads to survival of microbial flora in higher amounts at the site of the operation.

Intraoperative events may increase the risk in several ways, and these are also important factors:

- operative technique
- surgeon's skill
- duration of the operation
- break during the operation
- lack of asepsis.

The *operative technique* may inherit a certain risk that is characteristic of each type of operative procedure. Different operation techniques can be chosen at the same site to solve the same surgical problem. Differences can exist in the extent of tissue necrosis, vascular disturbance and blood retention, which are excellent 'mediums' for the growth of microbes. The type of closure – primary (tight) or secondary (loose), with or without a drain – is an important factor that may lead to dehiscence with consequent wound inflammation.

The *surgeon's skill* is thought to be an important factor, i.e. the ability to carry out the same type of operative technique in the shortest time with the least tissue damage, bleeding and necrosis. In surgeon's slang, it is called operating 'cleanly'. However, no two surgeons operate identically, which makes it difficult to study or prove this risk factor.

The *duration of the operation* can be a risk factor increasing the colonization level at the moment of closure and may decrease local defences through dryness and circulatory disturbance. This depends on the type of operation and on the surgeon's skill in carrying out the operation within an acceptable time according to the chosen method. Operations lasting more than two hours do not necessarily lead to higher risk.

A *break during an operation* prolongs the duration of the operation and may lead to injury asepsis. Any X-ray procedure above the wound can be critical.

Lack of any asepsis may lead to serious transmission of an infectious agent into the wound. It may be the result of an unskilled surgeon, a sterile or non-sterile nurse or just a lack of concentration during the operation. An instrument that is non-sterile for any reason is the most dangerous risk factor (see Chapter 5).

Postoperative wound care is a risk factor if it leads to delayed wound healing by not keeping the wound edges tight or by infecting the wound in any way (e.g. a non-sterile wound dressing).

The principle is that the closer the wound inflammation to the time of operation, the more likely it is that the inflammation process was induced during the operative procedure.

Prevention of wound infections

Prevention of wound infections may be achieved in several ways. Wound infection is one variety of HAI that can be prevented to a certain extent, but cannot be eliminated because of the presence of unavoidable risk factors. There are comprehensive guidelines and protocols (even duplicate published examples) giving instructions for preventing surgical wound infections (Garner et al., 1982; Garner, 1986; Kaiser, 1986; Mangram et al., 1999a, 1999b). The prevention strategy consists of three main elements:

- risk assessment of wound inflammation
- disease dose approach:
  - preparation of the wound site
  - aseptic operative process
  - antibiotic prophylaxis
  - aseptic wound care
- local defence mechanisms.

Risk assessment of wound inflammation is based on careful consideration of the benefits of the operation and the risk of any complications including wound inflammation. If the patient can be cured by methods other than an operation, the non-operative method should be used. Open traumatic wounds and vital indications are exceptions to this rule.

The *disease dose approach* consists of prevention by decreasing the microbial count in the wound, from endogenous and exogenous sources, to a level below the critical quantity if an operative procedure is indicated (see Figure 6.1).

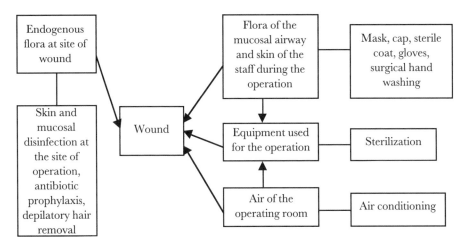

Figure 6.1. Sources of infectious agents in postoperative wound infections, and possible prevention.

Antibiotic prophylaxis does not replace other aseptic methods: preparation of operation site, sterilization of equipment that may come into direct or indirect contact with the wound, the behaviour of staff, and aseptic wound care (see Chapters 3 and 5).

Local defence mechanisms can be maintained only by the choice of the most gentle operation technique, and careful operative performance. To develop and to use appropriate surgical techniques is the task of surgery.

Pneumonia

Pneumonia is among the most frequent infections in both the community and hospitals. The lung is a vital organ that plays a role in the oxygen supply to the body and its functional impairment is one of the most frequent causes of death in hospitals.

Definition and diagnostic problems of pneumonia

Pneumonia is defined as inflammation of the lung (bronchioles, alveoli and interstitium). The diagnosis of pneumonia is one of the most difficult tasks because the lung is an internal organ and despite it being a cavity organ connected with the outer world by lower, middle and upper airways, there is no specific diagnostic method except for histology. In routine practice the clinical diagnosis and definition is clearly distinguished from the aetiological diagnosis, which relies mainly on the combination of three diagnostic methods whose sensitivity, specificity and predictive values, however, vary substantially:

- clinical diagnosis and definition:
  - clinical signs – cough, fever, pain, sputum, dyspnoea, auscultation of the lung
  - clinical laboratory test – leucocytosis, differential white blood cell analysis of the blood and sputum
  - X-ray – infiltrate
- aetiology – smear, culture of blood or airway exudate, molecular biology, serology.

The *clinical definition* of pneumonia is based on the clinical signs, laboratory tests and X-ray, while the microbiological methods – especially expectorated sputum culture – may help only to identify the aetiologic agent and does not necessarily confirm pneumonia. For the definition, it would be ideal to use a histopathological (biopsy or autopsy) diagnosis of the highest sensitivity and specificity, but transbronchial biopsy (TBB) or percutaneous lung biopsy (PLB) may induce serious complications, and autopsy is too late for the benefit of the patient.

However, clinical signs (except auscultation of the lung) and clinical laboratory tests are not specific to pneumonia because they may also be found in upper respiratory infections. The most difficult is to diagnose pneumonia in mechanically ventilated patients, where the clinical signs and the X-ray may be the same for other conditions: drug reaction, extrapulmonary infection and inflammation, blood transfusion, fibroproliferation, acute respiratory distress (ARDS), atelectasis, pulmonary embolism and haemorrhage, pleural effusion, congestive heart failure and tumour. Despite this, X-ray infiltrate is one of the most sensitive signs if carefully evaluated with other signs.

In *aetiological diagnosis* blood culture is useful together with clinical and radiographic methods if no other cause of microbemia can be found, but its sensitivity in finding the exact aetiology of the pneumonia is rather low because the microbemia cannot be caught in time in all cases.

Smear and culture of airway exudates may confirm the aetiology, but their predictive values depend on whether the identified microbe belongs to the normal oropharyngeal flora or not. Oropharyngeal flora may contaminate the sputum during the collection of the specimen, leading to false positive results. However, the presence of acid-fast bacilli (e.g. *Mycobacterium*) in the sputum confirms the diagnosis of tuberculosis (TB), thus remaining the gold standard in the rapid microbiological diagnosis of pulmonary TB despite its low sensitivity. Transbronchial collection of lower sputum has been developed in order to avoid contamination by oropharyngeal flora, assuming that a microbe in the lower respiratory tract is the cause of pneumonia. Bronchoscopy with bronchial washings (BW), bronchial brushings (BB), protected specimen brush (PSB) and bronchoalveolar lavage (BAL) have been utilized for this purpose (Baselski and Wunderink, 1994). However, the lower respiratory tract always contains microbes, which is why scientists have worked out quantitative culture methods using a diagnostic threshold to predict the aetiology of pneumonia. However, controversial views have been published concerning the predictive values of these methods, which confirms our diagnostic limitations (Baselski and Wunderink, 1994).

Serology confirms the aetiology in some infections, like those of viral origin (e.g. CMV and others) or *Mycoplasma pneumoniae* or *Chlamydia psittaci*, but its usefulness is limited in view of the lower occurrence of these microbes in the aetiology of pneumonia in the community and in hospitals, compared with other microbes.

Molecular biological methods are the latest to be used in the search for the aetiology of pneumonia, and they can be useful if other methods give false negative results, which may occur if the patient is under anti-microbial treatment at the time of the collection of the specimen. The highly sensitive polymerase chain reaction (PCR) has been implemented for diagnosis of TB by detecting *Mycobacterium*-specific genes in the sputum.

Aetiology and classification of pneumonia

Viruses, mycoplasmae, chlamydiae, bacteria, fungi or protozoa cause pneumonia, but their distribution varies in the community and in hospitals. The distribution of micro-organisms causing nosocomial pneumonia may be different in hospitals, owing to a difference in population and successful microbiological diagnosis. Different classification systems have been developed based on certain attributes:

- predisposing factors
- clinical-morphological
- acquisition of pneumonia.

Predisposing factors serve as a basis of classification, whether the pneumonia develops in the intact respiratory system or if there is a predisposing respiratory illness that precedes pneumonia. Two types are distinguished:

- primary pneumonia
- secondary pneumonia.

Primary pneumonia develops in an intact respiratory system and may be caused by any micro-organism. However, general resistance of humans may play a role in this type.

Secondary pneumonia occurs if there is a respiratory system disease other than pneumonia, which increases the risk of pneumonia. A chronic respiratory disease such as bronchial asthma or mucoviscidosis and others plays an important role. Mucoviscidosis is a predisposing factor for *Pseudomonas* infections.

The *clinical-morphological* classification was the first to be developed, classifying pneumonia into:

- typical
- atypical.

Typical pneumonia is mainly caused by *Streptococcus pneumoniae*, occurring mainly in the community, and in a severe form the inflammation is extended to a lobe of the lung (lobar pneumonia). This pneumonia is so characteristic of this germ that the shortened name is 'pneumococcus'. The pathological process involves the bronchioles, alveoli and interstitium and has well-defined consecutive phases. Clinically the onset is abrupt, then chills, fever, dyspnoea and a dry and productive purulent cough appear. Other micro-organisms such as *Haemophilus influenzae*, *Moraxella catarrhalis*, *Staphylococcus aureus*, *Klebsiella pneumoniae* may cause a similar clinical signs but the process remains in smaller foci not extending to a lobe (called subacute flow), and the phases of the infection are less characteristic so the pneumonia is usually called 'focal' rather than 'lobar'.

Atypical pneumonia differs both clinically and morphologically from the typical picture, with a milder flow, non-specific signs (fever, headache, myalgias), early non-productive cough, and scant and mucous sputum. The inflammation is restricted mainly to the interstitium, with less involvement of the alveoli and bronchioles. This type is usually caused by *Mycoplasmae*, *Chlamydiae*, *Coxiella*, *Pneumocystis carinii*, *Legionella spp.*, and viruses (varicella zoster, influenza, respiratory syncytial, etc.). It also occurs mainly in the community and is rare in hospital.

Acquisition of pneumonia is the third method of classification, though it should be emphasized that pneumonia cannot be acquired – only the infectious agent. This classification distinguishes two types, and has a strong rationale because the aetiology and the risk factors differ in many aspects:

- community-acquired pneumonia
- hospital-acquired pneumonia.

Community-acquired pneumonia (CAP) is mainly caused by the above-mentioned organisms (*Pneumococcus, Mycoplasmae, Haemophilus spp., Branchamella sp., Staphylococcus spp., Klebsiella spp., Legionella spp.*, and rarely by viruses such as the varicella zoster virus (in adults), cytomegalovirus (CMV), influenza virus, respiratory syncytial virus (RSV), etc.

Hospital-acquired pneumonia (HAP) is caused by a much wider range of micro-organisms than CAP. HAP is commonly divided into two main groups according to the appearance of pneumonia:

- early
- late.

Early HAP develops usually within five days after admission, and its aetiologic spectrum is almost the same as that for CAP, which confirms that the imported infectious agent causing the pneumonia began in hospital. This form should not be regarded as an imported CAI because the risk factors of being in hospital, such as mechanical ventilation or bronchoscopy, play a role in the induction of the pathological process. In the newborn, *Streptococcus agalactiae*, originating from the maternal flora, is the most frequent agent.

Late HAP usually develops after the fifth day following admission and the distribution of aetiologic agents is shifted to other micro-organisms than CAI. In late HAP, Gram-negative bacteria of *Pseudomonas spp., Acinetobacter spp.* and *Enterobacteriaceae*, and anaerobes (*Bacteroides spp.*) are the most frequent. Other bacteria also may occur, such as *Staphylococci* or *Enterococci*, but they are less frequent. In immunocompromised hosts fungi (*Aspergillus spp.*) occur quite often, and virus-induced (CMV) pneumonia in HIV patients can also be found.

HAP is further classified as to whether it is associated with mechanical ventilation or not. However, ventilation-associated pneumonia (VAP) is caused by the same micro-organism as other HAP; the difference lies only in the predisposing risk factors (Baselski and Wunderink, 1994).

Pathogenesis of pneumonia and sources of infection

In pneumonia, a micro-organism enters the lung (bronchioles, alveoli, and interstitium) and, by multiplying, causes inflammation of lung tissues, over-coming the host's clearing mechanisms from the nasal mucosa to the alveoli that act against the micro-organisms. The upper airway (nose and phar-ynx) filtrates and wets the air. Epiglottic and cough reflexes remove dust and microbes filtrated in the middle and lower airways or those gathering due to mucociliary transport by the epithelium of the trachea and bronchi. Mucociliary transport works like an escalator, where the inhaled particles impact on mucus covering the respiratory epithelium and the cilia project into the lower layer of mucus and beat in recurrent waves, propelling mucus and trapped particles upward to be expelled and swallowed (Mims et al., 2001, p. 21). In the alveolar clearance mechanism, the inhaled par-ticles reach the alveoli and are deposited on the surfactant layer. The alveo-lar macrophages phagocytize them and they migrate to the terminal bronchioles, where they are propelled upward to the mucociliary escalator. The cell-mediated and humoral immunity (secretory IgA) in the alveoli defeats microbes by killing them.

The deposition of particles in the respiratory tract depends on their diameter. Particles larger than 10 μm impact in the nasopharynx, those between 5 μm and 10 μm remain in the trachea, particles between 2 μm and 3 μm in diameter reach the bronchi, while only small particles of 1–2 μm impact in the bronchioles and alveoli. Breathing is a vital function to humans, thus exposure to microbes attached to the particles in the air happens every day and every minute of air. On average 400–900 micro-organisms are present per cubic metre of air, and therefore humans inhale 10 000 micro-organisms per day with a six litre per minute ventilation rate (Mims et al., 2001, p. 21). The lungs of newborns are pink in colour, but with ageing this changes to bluish-grey as a result of the deposit of particles in the interstitium, which cannot be cleared from the alveoli.

Without the respiratory defence mechanism, a human would develop at least one respiratory infection each day. Some micro-organisms may avoid being caught up in the mucus (through a defect in the layer), and resist the alveolar macrophages to reach and attach to the epithelium, causing disorder.

Infective agents may reach the lung by three mechanisms:

- bronchial
- haematogenous
- lymphatic vessels.

The *bronchial mechanism* in the development of pneumonia is the most common, and occurs by two means of pathomechanism:

- inhalation
- aspiration.

Inhalation brings into the lungs the infective agent from air that contains dust and droplets which harbour micro-organisms. Here the source of the infective agents is exogenous. This is the main mode of entry for *Aspergillus*, *Mycobacterium*, viruses, and some fungi both in the community and in hospitals. It is one of the modes of transmission between hosts of infectious agents called 'respiratory' infections (see Chapter 3). In the early 1960s, it was recognized that the unusual form of Gram-negative pneumonia was associated with inhalation therapy equipment in hospital intensive care units (Edmondson et al., 1966; Pierce et al., 1970; Sanders et al., 1970). Inhalation therapy equipment, which incorporates cold or heated *nebulizers*, frequently becomes colonized with Gram-negative bacteria and these are a source of infection. Different nebulizers are now used (such as ultrasonic, mainstream, medication, cascade, and paediatric isolettes) but their common feature is to achieve an adequate humidity of the air in the apparatus to avoid dryness of the respiratory tract. A container with cold water is an excellent medium for psychrophilic bacteria (*Pseudomonas spp.*, *Acinetobacter spp.*) that may grow in the nebulizer. Microaerosols created in the device transmit the infectious agents directly to the alveoli.

The infectious agent smallpox (variola virus), the pulmonary form of plague (*Yersinia pestis*) and anthrax (*Bacillus anthracis*) are all acquired through inhalation. These may become tools for bio-terrorism. The difference between them is that the agent of anthrax does not spread between humans, while plague and smallpox can be transmitted. Furthermore, *Legionella spp.* is a dangerous agent if it colonizes air-conditioning systems causing outbreaks both in the community and in hospitals (Eickhoff, 1979).

Aspiration is a common mechanism whereby the micro-organism reaches the lung with aspirated fluid from the oropharynx or through the regurgitation of the contents of the stomach. Micro-aspiration (when a small quantity of fluid is aspired) happens in almost every healthy human, but macro-aspiration (when a large quantity is aspired) is an important mechanism, occurring both in CAP and in HAP. The macro-aspiration occurs when an unconscious patient vomits and the aspirate is so large that even the normal respiratory defence is not able to clear the airways. The second mode occurs if the clearing reflexes in the pharynx are disturbed for any reason and cannot remove even small quantities of aspirate. The third type occurs when an endotracheal tube is inserted into the trachea and aspiration occurs alongside the tube from leakage around the cuff in mechanically ventilated patients, even for a short period (narcosis, or ventilation up to 48 hours) or in the case of long-term ventilation (more than 48 hours). Any micro-organism colonizing the aspirate may cause pneumonia if it reaches the distal part of the lung. Aerobic and anaerobic bacteria and fungi play a role in this mechanism.

In the aspiration mechanism, the infectious agent may originate from an endogenous source (nasopharynx, gastric colonization, paranasal sinuses), which is usually called the 'endogenous reservoir', or it may come from an exogenous source when the nasopharynx of the patient is manipulated by an instrument (nasogastric or orogastric tube, bronchosopy, gastroscopy) or by a human hand (oral toilette).

The *haematogenous spread* of micro-organisms may occur from a distant endogenous focus of the infectious process. The process is often called 'septic embolization', where the microbes attached to the emboli reach the lung via the venous system flowing from the organs where the primary infection occurs. Thus, pneumonia may follow any type of bloodstream infection, but bacterial sepsis is the main cause of this spread. However, viruses such as cytomegalovirus in an immunocompromised host (HIV, bone marrow transplants, etc.) may also cause pneumonia via this pathway.

Lymphatic vessels may transport micro-organisms to the lung from the abdomen and lower extremities because of anatomical features of the lymphatic vessels. However, this type of spread is difficult to verify because of the difficulties of culturing the lymph.

Risk factors for pneumonia

A variety of papers have been published to define all the possible risk factors for HAP. However, this is a most difficult task because of the problem of exact clinical and aetiological diagnosis, especially in ventilated patients, and the concurrent occurrence of pneumonia with other forms of HAI. More than 20 risk factors have been evaluated and among them the strongest risk factors appear to be mechanical ventilation or tracheal intubation, which can be explained by the differences in pathogenetic factors.

According to the pathogenesis, all the possible endogenous and exogenous risk factors may be grouped into three categories, which corresponds to the concept of disease dose (see Chapter 2):

* dose and/or pathogenicity of the micro-organism inoculated
* decreased local respiratory clearance
* impaired systemic immunity.

The *dose and/or pathogenicity of the micro-organism* must be increased in order to achieve the disease dose (DD). We have to bear in mind that pathogenicity is relative, thus the DD may be altered by both the virulence of the micro-organism and the defence of the host (see Chapter 2). The limit of DD may be reached by two mechanisms:

* increased frequency and/or the volume of aspiration
* inhalation mode.

Increased aspiration encompasses risk factors such as unconsciousness, nasoenteric tube, upper abdominal surgery and endotracheal ventilation, where the dose of infectious agent is increased purely by the increased volume of the aspirate (macroaspirate), which cannot be cleared completely even by a healthy respiratory tract.

Inhalation should not be increased if the microbe is virulent enough to cause pneumonia. However, the dose of viable microbes per unit of inhaled air must also reach the DD. Air conditioning with an increased quantity of microbes and the ventilation of patients with infected nebulizers belong to this group.

Decreased respiratory clearance is the second main risk category. When existing clearance mechanisms are disturbed, or when sedation is used, they are not able to clear the microaspirates. In chronic lung diseases, unconsciousness, use of sedatives, narcosis and endotracheal ventilation, clearance by the nasopharynx does not function, so the risk is increased. The endotracheal tube may cause mechanical irritation of airways which may also cause decreased functionality.

Impaired systemic immunity has also been mentioned as a risk factor, but is not specific to pneumonia. Among the factors, age, poor nutritional state and hypoalbuminaemia have been described. Here the mechanism can be the overall decrease of immunity leading to decreased local defence of the lung, but the role of the latter has not been isolated.

It seems that the most frequent risk factors are: mechanical ventilation, chronic lung disease, severity of the illness, age, severe head trauma, and depressed level of consciousness.

Prevention of pneumonia

The prevention strategy for pneumonia has several intervention points. However, the effectiveness may vary depending on the ability to influence the risk factors from among the many that may occur in an individual.

One prevention strategy, when the pneumonia is vaccine preventable, is the use of vaccines. There are vaccines against the 'b' type of *Haemophylus infuenzae* (Hib), the influenza virus, the varicella zoster virus and several stereotypes of *Pneumococcus*. At first glance it seems that their main use is against CAP while not influencing the occurrence of HAP, where the aetiology is shifted to the Gram-negative bacteria and fungi against which no vaccine has been developed. However, it is not logical to separate the preventive strategies for CAP and HAP. The reason is that patients with severe CAP are admitted to hospital and need further invasive procedures including puncture of the chest (for empyema) or even mechanical ventilation, because the oxygenization of the body is decreased due to the severity of CAP. This may lead to super-infection of existing CAP by hospital flora, which maintains the pneumonia in the patient. It should be noted that the most common complication and cause of death through influenza in old people (aged 60 years plus) is *Pneumococcus* pneumonia. Thus, vaccination against influenza and *Pneumococcus* is indicated for this age group.

If pneumonia is *not* preventable by vaccines, the strategy depends on the development mechanism of pneumonia, and whether the potential source of the infectious agent is exogenous (inhalation, aspiration) or endogenous (aspiration, haematogenous, lymphatic vessels) or both. Here non-specific preventive measures should be used (see Chapter 5).

- exogenous and inhalation mechanisms:
  - protective isolation of the susceptible person (especially if immuno-compromised, e.g. organ transplantation, etc.):
    - single-bedded room
    - mask for those who may shed any infectious agent from the respiratory tract
  - cleaning and disinfection of the air-conditioning system and filtering of the air

- mechanical ventilation:
  - sterilization of the nebulizer
  - sterile water must be used to humidify in the nebulizer
  - change of breathing circuits
  - avoid opening the patient's mechanical ventilation system; if this is necessary, sterile gloves should be used
- source is exogenous and aspiration mechanism:
  - manipulation in the oropharynx of the patient:
    - sterile gloves;
    - sterile medical equipment
  - sterile endotracheal tube
- source is endogenous:
  - prevention of vomiting
  - prevention of aspiration by positioning the head in an appropriate elevated position
  - oral hygiene with mucosal disinfectant
  - preservation of the acidity of the stomach
  - orogastric tubes instead or nasogastric tubes
  - frequently sucking the leakage in mechanical ventilation.

There are written guidelines recommending the above measures (Tablan et al., 1994a, 1994b). Some scientists accept some preventive action as ritual and claim to have undertaken well-designed observational or experimental epidemiological studies. However, for ethical and other reasons it is impossible to conduct such studies, and so preventive actions are accepted for logical reasons. It should be emphasized that all the above mentioned measures are in accordance with the concept of the transmission and disease dose as fundamentals in infectious disease development (see Chapter 2 and Chapter 3). The more mechanisms that are involved in the development of an infectious disease the more difficult it is to prevent the disease. HAP falls into this category.

Gastrointestinal infections

Gastrointestinal infections are among the most frequent nosocomial infections in both developed and developing countries. Their occurrence and causative profile vary among countries, type of health care institutions and patient populations. Gastroenteric infections are easily controllable, although they may occur as sporadic cases, in clusters or even as outbreaks (Stamm et al., 1981; Levine et al., 1991).

Definition and classification of gastrointestinal infections

Gastrointestinal infections (GI) can be defined as the disorders of the stomach and intestines (small and large bowel) that have an infectious origin. However, the gastrointestinum is only part of the alimentary tract, and infection of parts other than the gastrointestinum, such as the oral cavity, oesophagus and rectum, may occur. However, their pathogenesis and risk factors usually differ from gastrointestinal infections affecting the stomach and bowel system.

GIs are classified according to the main location of the infection and clinical symptoms, but different parts may be affected at the same time:

* gastritis (stomach) – vomiting and nausea, pain in the upper abdomen
* enteritis (small bowel) – passage of a few voluminous stools or watery diarrhoea, abdominal pain
* colitis (large bowel) – passage of many small-volume stools, bloody diarrhoea, tenesmus, pain in lower abdomen.

Diarrhoea is the common symptom of both enteritis and colitis, and in many instances all parts of the bowel are involved, when it is called enterocolitis. If vomiting and diarrhoea exist the process involves both the stomach and small bowel (gastroenteritis). Fever is the sign of a severe form, which is due to the production of toxin.

In defining hospital-acquired gastrointestinal infections (HAGI) two critical points should be taken into account:

* Clinical signs of gastorenteritis are non-specific, thus proper differential diagnosis is needed to discriminate between infectious and non-infectious causes (toxicoses, parasympathomimetic agents, cardiovascular medications, antimetabolites, osmotic cathartics, antacids, hyperalimentation preparations, pancreatic islet tumours, carcinoid tumours, hypoparathyroidism, diabetes, gastrointestinal cancer, uraemia, blind loop syndromes colonic mass, or lesions) (McFarland, 1993). However, diarrhoea can be a clinical sign of severe sepsis. The presence of microorganisms in the stools is a requirement for the infectious origin of gastrointestinal infections; however, microbiological methods often fail to detect in the faeces any microbes responsible for the diarrhoea.
* Hospital acquisition of an infectious agent, or hospital factors inducing the development of symptoms, must be considered. The period between admission and the onset of symptoms, previous antibiotic treatment and

careful epidemiological analysis, together with the microbiological results, serve to distinguish community-acquired GI (CAGI) from hospital acquired GI. The term 'nosocomial diarrhoea' has been introduced (though is not the best suggestion); if the symptoms begin 72 hours or later after admission it is recognized as hospital-acquired. However, the incubation period of individual micro-organisms should be taken into account, and the 72-hour cut-off point may be accepted only for GI of undefined aetiology.

The GI can be classified into two main groups:

- manifest:
  - food-borne intoxications
  - gastroenterocolitis
  - malabsorption
- inapparent.

Food-borne intoxications are caused by oral intake of different toxins produced by an infectious agent pre-existing in food if appropriate conditions are present (genetic code and ability to produce toxins, temperature). The time needed for toxin production is called the 'external incubation' period. Here the disease dose (DD) is determined by the quantity of toxin per unit of food, and the quantity of microbial particles is secondary. However, additional growth in the bowel (e.g. *Salmonella spp.*, or *Shigella spp.*) may occur in food-borne intoxications as the result of ingestion of viable microbial particles.

Gastroenterocolitis occurs if the infectious agent grows in the alimentary tract, achieving the DD and overwhelming the host defences, causing different types of inflammatory processes. Humans may further spread the agent into the environment via stools.

Malabsorption occurs as a result of the decreased absorption of nutrients owing to gastrointestinal infections, or shortage of nutrients because the infectious agent takes them up (e.g. Giardia lamblia, intestinal worms).

Causes and pathogenesis of gastrointestinal infections

A wide range of micro-organisms may cause gastrointestinal infections: viruses, bacteria, intestinal protozoa and helminths. Pathogenesis and causes of GI are associated and present a characteristic clinical picture.

Gastritis develops due to the intake of a large amount of toxin produced by the infectious agent or local growth of *Helicobacter pylori*.

Diarrhoea develops by three mechanisms:

- increased motility of the bowel
- increased secretion of water through the wall of the bowel
- decreased reabsorption of water in the large bowel.

Infectious agents mainly cause diarrhoea by the increased secretion of water by toxin production causing diarrhoea and/or adherence to the mucosa of the bowel, causing three main processes:

- adherence to mucosa without invasion and toxin production, causing inflammation or haemorrhagia
- invasion of the agent with an intense inflammatory response by cell death
- enterotoxin production stimulating the intracellular cyclic adenosine-monophosphate (cAMP) leading to increased active secretion, leaving the mucosa intact.

Gastroenteritis is mainly characteristic of food-borne intoxications caused by *Bacillus cereus* and enterotoxin-producing strains of *Staphylococcus aureus*, *Salmonella spp.* or *Shigella spp.* Viruses such as rotavirus or Norwalk virus also cause gastroenteritis involving the stomach and invading the small bowel. Isolated gastritis is caused by *Helicobacter pylori*, which play a role in haemorrhagic gastritis and ulcerative disease of the stomach.

Diarrhoea of small bowel origin by cAMP activation is caused by *Vibrio cholerae*, *Giardia lamblia* or enterotoxigenic *Escherichia coli* (ETEC). Adhered agent toxins can also affect the small bowel – ETEC, by enteropathogenic *Escherichia coli* (EPEC) or *Shigella spp.* (early phase), while invasion occurs by *Salmonella spp.*, or enteroinvasive *Escherichia coli* (EIEC). *Salmonella spp.* may reach distant organs such as the lung or bones, causing a wide range of invasive *Salmonella* infections.

Diarrhoea of large bowel origin may be caused by mucosal invasion of *Shigella spp.*, *Campylobacter jejuni*, *Entamoeba histolytica*. Large bowel mesenteric lymphangitis is usually caused by *Yersinia enterocolitica*, and can be confused with appendicitis. The toxin 'A' of *Clostridium difficile* may damage the large bowel, causing pseudomembranous colitis, which is a serious consequence of an antibiotic treatment. Here the mechanism is the death of normal bowel flora and overgrowth of *C. difficile*, thus this type of diarrhoea is also called 'antibiotic-associated colitis' to distinguish it from other causes. It is quite common and mainly occurs as HAI. All patients receiving antibiotic treatment who develop diarrhoea are suspected of having the *C. difficile* infection.

There is one infection, caused by toxins of *Clostriduim botulinum*, which instead of gastroenterocolitis causes neurological symptoms (dysarthria, dysphagia, diplopia), but this infection occurs via food. Toxins of *C. botulinum* may be used for bioterrorism.

In the case of protozoal infection caused by *Giardia lamblia*, the agent covers the mucosa of the small bowel, inhibiting the absorption of nutrients. Chronic mild diarrhoea may occur (see above). Another mechanism of malabsorption occurs when the large intestinal helminths such as *Taenia saginata*, *Taenia solium* or *Ascaris lumbricoides* take up nutrients from the host.

Source of the infectious agent in gastrointestinal infections

Sources of infectious agents of the alimentary tract are always exogenous with the exception of antibiotic-associated colitis, where the *C. difficile* may originate from endogenous or exogenous sources (McFarland et al., 1989). Sources can be human only (*Shigella spp.*, *Staphylococcus aureus*, *Salmonella typhi*, *Giardia lamblia*, *Entamoeaba histolytica*, etc.) or both human and animal (other *Salmonella spp.*, *Campylobacter jejuni*, *Yesinia enterocolitica*) or animal only (e.g. *Taenia saginata*). An inanimate environment such as soil (*Clostridium botulinum*) may also serve as a source. Water, food, hand or endoscopes inserted into the alimentary tract can serve as vehicles for the transmission of infectious agents (O'Connor and Axon, 1983; Alvarado et al., 1991).

Risk factors of nosocomial gastrointestinal infections

Among endogenous risk factors, decreased stomach acidity is one of the most common. Newborns, and adults taking antacids (sodium bicarbonate, H_2-blockers,) are at increased risk due to low stomach acidity. The change of bowel flora (antibiotic treatment) is another factor. Both types of risk factor lead to the lower level of disease dose required for the development of GI.

Endoscopic procedures are regarded as exogenous risk factors, when infectious agents may be transmitted between patients as a result of inappropriate cleaning and disinfection (O'Connor and Axon, 1983; Alvarado et al., 1991). Microbes in the inserted endoscope evade the stomach acid thus providing an attachment primarily to the bowel, where the pH is close to neutral.

Prevention of nosocomial gastrointestinal infections

The prevention strategy for GI (intoxication or gastroenterocolitis) depends on the possible source of the infectious agent and whether the infectious agent can be transmitted from humans by any means or not. All gastrointestinal infections follow the 'faecal–oral' mechanisms of the transmission of infectious agents, which can be direct or indirect (see Chapter 3 and McFarland, 1993).

Any raw animal material used for nutritional purposes should be considered as a potential source of infectious agents, thus appropriate cooking is the most essential element in the prevention of food-borne infections, both intoxication and gastroenteritis. All parts of the meal need cooking for a minimum of ten minutes at 100°C. Control of the catering service and the prevention of recontamination of cooked food are further steps in the interruption of the transmission of an infectious agent.

As humans are a source of infectious agents they may shed the agent into the environment through faeces, and if it contaminates water, food or the hand, it may be transmitted further. The hand serves as a vehicle where a low disease dose causes clinical infection, as in the case of *Shigella* where only 100 viable particles are necessary. Food and water are needed to achieve a higher dose, as for *Salmonella spp.*, which requires more than 1000 particles. Water sanitation and personal hygiene with appropriate hand washing are an essential element in the prevention of GIs, and also an important measure for the self-defence of medical staff.

Cleaning and appropriate disinfection of all equipment contaminated with faeces is an important factor in the prevention of hospital-acquired GIs. Use and appropriate changing of gloves decreases the probability of the transmission of infectious agents if such equipment should be touched.

Bloodstream infections

Bloodstream infections are among the top ten hospital-acquired infections in both developed and developing countries. This is connected with increased invasive procedures in health care.

Definition and types of bloodstream infections

Bloodstream infection is defined as the presence and growth of a microorganism in the blood. This term should not be confused with the term 'blood-borne infection' because the latter means only that the infectious agent is transmitted via the blood. In blood-borne infections, the blood serves as the portal of entry or exit for the microbe in the chain of transmission between hosts (see Chapter 3). For some infectious agents, the blood serves not only as the portal of entry or exit, but also as a place of primary habitat; for example: HIV in T4-lymphocytes or *Plasmodia* multiplying in the red blood cells, causing malaria. For others, blood serves *only* as the portal of entry or exit because the microbe grows in other tissues (e.g. hepatitis B virus). Some micro-organisms, especially bacteria and fungi, may attach to the endocardium of the heart, causing endocarditis leading to intermittent or continuous spreading of the agents into the blood. However, inflammation of veins or arteries may also occur due to the spreading. Microbes may also attach to emboli causing pulmonary emboli or 'septic emboli' in organs, depending on the direction of spread.

The outcome of bloodstream infections can be various, and two forms are distinguished according to the host's reaction:

- microbemia
- sepsis.

Microbemia is the presence of a micro-organism in the blood without a systemic reaction of the host, and the type of the microbe is specified (viremia, bacteremia, fungemia, protozonemia, etc.). It can be inapparent or it may be followed by non-specific clinical symptoms (fever, low-grade temperature, fatigue, weakness, shivering). The duration of microbemia is of importance in identifying the source and the need for treatment, which can be:

- transient
- sustained or continuous
- intermittent.

Transient microbemia lasts several minutes, and it occurs in bacterial pneumonia, meningitis and pyelonephritis, but may occur in chewing, tooth brushing or instrumentation.

Sustained or continuous microbemia lasts several hours or days, indicating a permanent source of the microbe in the body, and is usually intravascular (infected artery, vein, heart valve, or shunt) or extravascular (abscess, extravascular device or other focus) for bacterial and fungal infections.

Intermittent microbemia occurs if the microbe is shedding intermittently into the blood.

Microbemia can be limited in time or even lifelong (e.g. HIV) depending on the natural flow of the infectious process in an individual.

Sepsis is a form of bloodstream infection; its definition is still disputable, being without consensus despite many attempts to provide a uniform definition (Balk and Bone, 1989; Ackerman 1994; Bone, 1994, 1996; Karzai and Reinhart, 1998; Fry, 2000). The main distinction between sepsis and a simple microbemia is that sepsis induces a well-distinguished *systemic reaction* in the host, which is not characteristic of microbemia. Most experts agree that sepsis syndrome, recently called systemic inflammatory response syndrome (SIRS), consists of disturbed thermoregulation (fever or hypothermia), tachypnea, tachycardia, reduced vascular resistance, leukocytosis or leukopenia, and evidence of impaired organ perfusion. However, the term SIRS is used for non-infectious mechanisms such as inflammation by injury, shock, severe tissue damage and inflammation (Bone, 1994, 1996; Fry, 2000). Intensive research to find other parameters specific to infectious SIRS, for example plasma procalcitonin level, is ongoing. The presence of infection leading to sepsis syndrome lies in the differentiation of infectious from non-infectious SIRS.

Septic shock is the severest form of sepsis, leading to death in more than 60% of cases due to multi-organ failure because of decreased perfusion. It is sepsis if systolic blood pressure is less than 90 mm Hg or there is a reduction of at least 40 mm Hg.

Multiple organ dysfunction syndrome (MODS) is impaired organ function due to decreased perfusion requiring intervention.

Pathogenesis, sources and the aetiology of bloodstream infections

The pathogenesis, the source and the expected micro-organism of bloodstream infections are correlated with each other. As stated in Chapter 2, blood connects all organs via circulation in blood vessels, and infectious agents may spread by means of blood circulation from one focus to another. However, the common feature of all types of bloodstream infections is that the infectious agent should pass through the skin and mucosal barrier to reach the vascular system. Based on transmission concepts, bloodstream infections can be further classified as:

- primary
- secondary
- mixed.

The mechanism of bloodstream infection depends on whether it is primary or secondary. These two forms have different implications for infection control practice and therapeutic management. Mixed types follow the characteristics of both the primary and secondary types.

Primary bloodstream infections are those in which the infectious agent localizes primarily in the blood without a related infection at another site (Garner et al., 1988). This requires that an *exogenous source* should provide the microbe, which can be mainly viruses (HIV), or protozoa (e.g. *Plasmodia*). Transient microbemia from an endogenous source does not fall into this category. This type of bloodstream infection – except HIV and malaria – is rare in hospitals (Garfield et al., 1978). The Centers for Disease Control (CDC) has classified intravascular device-associated bloodstream infections as primary even if the infection is present at the site of access (Garner et al., 1988). However, classifying such infections as primary is not the best choice because it leads to a classification overlap that may cause confusion. In primary bloodstream infections, the agent invades the host in one of three ways:

- natural invasiveness
- biological vector (e.g. mosquito) provides inoculation
- intravascular procedures:
    - temporary devices:
        - intravascular catheters
        - intravenous injection with metallic needles
    - permanent devices:
        - implants
    - intravenous blood products and medication.

In primary bloodstream infection, no extravascular foci of the infection are found in the host. Very few microbes have natural invasiveness (spirilla, spirochetes). In the community, mosquitoes serve to inoculate the *Plasmodia*, while non-sterile syringes and needles are common vehicles in the transmission of HIV in community drug users. In hospitals, *non-sterile* intravascular devices (intravascular catheters monitoring blood gas and haemodynamic parameters, collection of blood for laboratory analysis, prosthetic valves) are important mechanisms of inoculation from exogenous sources, or if the intravenous or blood product is contaminated (Maki et al., 1976).

Secondary bloodstream infections have an *extravascular endogenous* focus with the same microbe being in the blood. The infectious agent grows in the endogenous source and the agent is injected into the blood. For example, wound infection caused by *Staphylococci*, or *Escherichia coli* causing pyelonephritis may spread further and cause infection in other organs. Two types of endogenous sources of secondary bloodstream infections can be distinguished:

- normal microbial flora consisting of bacteria and fungi
- primary infection in an organ.

The role of normal microbial flora containing different micro-organisms in different parts of the body is extremely important in hospital-acquired bloodstream infections. The main cause of bloodstream infections depends on which part of the body serves as the source of the infection (see Chapter 1 and Table 1.9). If the endogenous source is an infected organ then any type of micro-organism can be expected. Secondary bloodstream infections may develop as a result of two main mechanisms:

- natural invasiveness
- extravascular invasive procedures:
    - temporary device:
        ○ drains
        ○ catheters
        ○ operations
    - permanent device:
        ○ implants.

The *natural invasiveness* leads to bloodstream infections from the endogenous primary focus in the host, which is the result of the natural invasiveness of a micro-organism. Any kind of organ may serve as a primary focus, especially cavity organs with a gate to the outer world (paranasal sinuses, gall bladder, urogenital tract etc.). Such infections are usually community acquired, but hospital acquisition may also occur. Others, like hepatitis B and C viruses, replicate in the liver and spread into the blood. As mentioned above, the blood is a secondary habitat for these microbes.

Extravascular invasive procedures are the most common mechanism of secondary hospital-acquired bloodstream infections due to the high risk of infection and the high prevalence of invasive procedures on different organs in hospitals. Any invasive procedure or operation – even without leaving any foreign body in the host – may cause bloodstream infection where the microbe originates from the site of the invasive procedure.

Mixed bloodstream infection occurs if the source of the infectious agent can be both endogenous and exogenous. Many invasive device-associated bloodstream infections follow this pattern, sharing the features of both primary and secondary bloodstream infections. Intravascular catheter-associated bloodstream infections also fall into this category: medication or the infusion can be contaminated, or a person's hand may infect the catheter as an exogenous source, while the skin at the point of insertion of the catheter or the infected tunnel serves as endogenous source.

All devices provoke a reaction in the host, which tries to cover the foreign body with fibronectin and other substances, which in turn serve as receptors for the attachment of microbes to the device. Some devices are left in the host for a few minutes or days (catheters, drains) while others (implants) are lifelong (e.g. hip prosthesis). The device can serve as a source for secondary bloodstream infection until it is removed. However, with permanent devices it is desirable to leave the implant lifelong in order to promote the function of that organ where it is inserted.

The infectious agent may reach the blood at two stages in any type of device-associated bloodstream infection:

- insertion of the device
- maintenance.

For those devices that have no external access through the skin or mucosa (such as a prosthetic heart valve) after insertion the infection occurs mainly at the stage of insertion from an exogenous and/or endogenous source at the site of operation. Usually *Staphylococci* are the leading cause. If the infection happens at the stage of maintenance then it can develop only by the haematogenous or lymphatic spread of a microbe from distant organs with consequent attachment to the implant. In many situations, an exacerbation of early inapparent infection occurs.

If the device has an external access through the skin or mucosa during its period of functioning then infection may also occur on insertion and/or maintenance, but the difference is that the source of the infectious agent can be endogenous and/or exogenous at the stage of maintenance. Microbes may colonize the site of access, invading the host on the external surface of the device.

Prevention of bloodstream infections

A variety of scientific papers have been published on the prevention of bloodstream infections, especially intravascular catheter-associated infections (Maki et al., 1987; Dickinson and Bisno, 1989a, 1989b). Several organizations have published complex revised guidelines, sometimes in duplicate (Pearson et al., 1996a, 1996b; Mermel et al., 2001a, 2001b).

The basis of prevention strategies for bloodstream infections is the transmission concept, just as for other infections. The aim of prevention is to interrupt the transmission of infectious agents from endogenous and exogenous sources to the bloodstream. Additionally, device-dependence, with or without external access, should be taken into account.

If the source is exogenous and no intravascular procedure occurs (natural invasiveness, vector-borne) then control is restricted to the community (control of HIV among sexually active persons, malaria control by anti-malarial drugs, etc.).

If the source of the infectious agent is exogenous, and an intravascular and/or extravascular invasive procedure is carried out, the following measures are necessary:

- insertion of the device:
    - sterilization of inserted device (syringe, needle, catheter, valve, implant, etc.) before insertion
    - sterile medication (injection, infusion solutions)
    - avoidance of contamination (aseptic circumstances) during insertion:
        ○ sterile gloves
        ○ mask during insertion
        ○ sterile coat if the insertion occurs in operating room
- screening the blood product for agents that can be transmitted e.g. HIV, hepatitis B and C, prions, cytomagalovirus, viruses causing malignancy, *Plasmodia*, etc.
- maintenance of the device if there is an external access:
    - aseptic manipulation (sterile gloves)
    - disinfection of the device left outside the body
    - closed drainage system, but disinfection if it should be open.

If the source of the infectious agent is endogenous then the following measures are needed:

- if an intravasular and/or extravascular invasive procedure is done:
    - insertion of device:
        ○ avoiding insertion at the site where infection has occurred
        ○ skin or mucosal disinfection at the site of insertion
    - maintenance of the device if there is an external access:
        ○ disinfection at the site of access preventing colonization

- replacement of the infected device:
- if no preliminary invasive procedures are done:
  - search for primary focus of infection in different extravascular organs
  - elimination of extravascular foci of infection by:
    - surgical treatment
    - antibiotic treatment.

Summary

This chapter focuses on the most frequent forms of hospital-acquired infections. The following points must be emphasized:

- The transmission concept is a common feature of infections regardless of whether they are hospital acquired or not.
- Invasive procedures may cause infection from both endogenous and exogenous sources.
- Other infections, such as infections of the central nervous system, eyes, ear–nose–pharynx, etc., follow the same principles as wound infections if invasive procedures are carried out on these organs.
- The principles are the same if the agent originates from an endogenous source, where the type of expected colonization flora depends on the site of entry, or from an exogenous source, which depends on the transmission characteristics of the particular infectious agent.
- Unfortunately, it is almost impossible to eliminate the endogenous source of patients, which explains the limitations of the prevention of HAI from such sources.
- The general principle of prevention of all device-associated infections is that a device should be used only when necessary and should be removed as soon as possible.
- Prevention of bloodstream infections in hospitals is a most complex problem, because it depends on the prevention of extravascular infections as well.

CHAPTER 7

Infection control and surveillance

Hospital epidemiology and clinical microbiology – basic principles

Epidemiology is the study of the distribution and determinants of health-related states or events in a specified population (Last, 1995 p. 55). The word *epidemiology* is of Greek origin: *epidemo(s)* from *epi* = on + *demos* = the people, meaning 'among people' (Churchill's, 1989, p. 627).

Epidemiology is one of the youngest of the sciences but its methods were used in the nineteenth century for infectious diseases long before the formulation of its general theory (Semmelweis, 1861; Langmuir, 1976). The renaissance of epidemiology occurred with the need to standardize the general methods of seeking causes of diseases.

Epidemiology uses two distinct methods:

* descriptive
* analytical.

Descriptive epidemiology describes the occurrence of disease by frequency distribution, comparing different populations, and/or different times, and/or different places, thereby formulating a hypothesis about the causes of the disease. It answers the questions: Who is at risk? When does it occur? Where does it occur? What are the possible causes and determinants?

Analytical epidemiology searches for causes by estimating the probability of associations between determinants and health events, and by testing statistical hypotheses it answers the questions: Why and how does the health event develop? How strong is the association between the determinants and health event?

The aim of the health care process in hospitals is to restore the normal physiological state of humans. In this process, human (medical staff and technical staff) and technical resources are involved in achieving the final goal. The concept of 'quality of health care' has been developed to assess and monitor the health care systems (Donabedian, 1978). However, both infectious and non-infectious complications can occur, and these are the negative indicators of the quality of the health care system (see Figure 7.1).

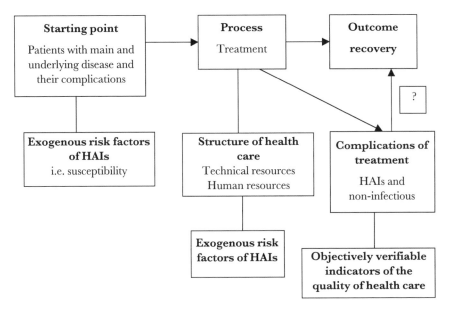

Figure 7.1. Structure of health care and its relation to HAI.

The professional, legal and economic problems associated with these complications, and the specific characteristics of the hospital population, have led to the development of *hospital epidemiology* with the aim of decreasing such events (see Figure 7.2).

Hospital epidemiology was born in the nineteenth century when Ignacz Semmelweis in 1861 published his book *The Etiology, Concept and Prophylaxis of Childbed Fever*, analysing scientifically the determinants of childbed fever in the Maternity Hospital of Vienna (Semmelweis, 1861).

Hospital epidemiology in the twentieth century became part of infection control in hospitals, contributing to the quality of health care (see Figure 7.3). It promotes infection control, using the methods mentioned above.

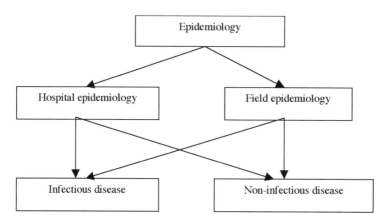

Figure 7.2. Main divisions of epidemiology by the two main disease patterns and population investigated.

The aims of infection control in hospitals

The aims of the control of HAIs are the same as in general epidemiology:

- The *primary* aim of prevention is to discover all the determinants that influence the occurrence and magnitude of the health event of interest (Beaglehole et al., 1993, p. 88). It means to 'know' what lies behind the natural process of the infection and to know its 'behaviour' in the population under investigation. If the preventive measures lead to a decrease in occurrence it means that the infection is under human control.
- The *secondary* aim is to prevent disability or death by early diagnosis and effective treatment avoiding the complication of the health event itself (Beaglehole et al., 1993, p. 91). The prompt treatment of an infection – especially of severe infections like sepsis – serves the further prevention of other infections in the same patient, so avoiding further invasive procedures and promoting early discharge.

Organization of infection control

The prevention of HAI requires the organization, establishment and promotion of measures by the hospital administration. These may also be regulated by national laws. However, legal enforcement is usually less effective than voluntary-based infection control.

Throughout the world the infection control of HAI has become an independent medical discipline since it was first recognized in the USA during

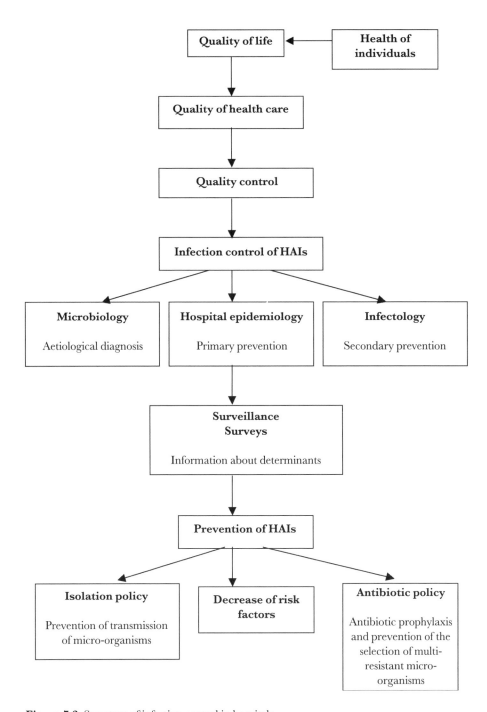

Figure 7.3. Structure of infection control in hospitals.

the 1960s as being an essential part of the quality control of health care in hospitals (see Figure 7.3). In many countries there is also a requirement for the audit of hospitals by health care accreditation programmes (Donabedian, 1978). The aim of such audits is the permanent improvement of the quality of health care by means of regular revision of the existing systems, which also applies to infection control. Another reason for audits is that the economic resources in hospitals are limited, and their use needs planning and continuous evaluation.

An infection control system cannot be effective unless it follows all the systems inplace. The system is evaluated to discover whether all the human and technical conditions exist in order to achieve the appropriate outcome with minimal complications (see Figure 7.1). The audit process evaluates whether the available resources are being used properly. Any changes to the system will result in changes in the outcome, with changes in the frequency of complications being the indicator.

The control of HAI consists of two distinct parts:

- the 'controlled part', which is composed of the *'patient–structure–process'* elements of health care (see Figure 7.1)
- the 'controlling part' organizing the control policy and processes, which consists of the *'microbiology–epidemiology–infectology'* elements, observing health care in hospital, and evaluating the function and outcomes of the controlled part (see Figure 7.3):
  - Microbiology provides the diagnostic element of HAI, confirming the aetiology for the case definition and enabling effective treatment by measuring the anti-microbial resistance of the infectious agent.
  - Epidemiology deals with primary prevention by designing preventive strategies against HAI.
  - Infectology serves the treatment of HAI by providing a secondary means of prevention.

In the process of infection control, the controlled and controlling parts play different roles. In rare situations they are not separated, thus establishing self-control. This happened in the work of Semmelweis when he combined the role of both functions at the same time (Semmelweis, 1861).

Conflicts may arise between these two parts, especially when the importance of infection control is ignored by the controlled part. Voluntary recognition of the problem of HAI is a key issue.

Personnel requirements for infection control in hospitals

Successful infection control needs well-trained controlling staff to organize the process. In most hospitals it is the Infection Control Committee (ICC) that organizes the strategy and policy. It consists of:

- *essential members*: a member of the hospital management, director of nursing, microbiologist, infectologist (clinical microbiologist), hospital epidemiologist, pharmacist, supplies manager, sterile supply manager, manager of the cleaning department, representative of clinical staff
- *additional members*: a member from the engineering department, and voluntary members from the clinical departments.

The task of the ICC is to formulate the strategy of infection control via regular meetings at which it considers different policies, programmes and local documents on infection control.

The Infection Control Team (ICT) is responsible for the day-to-day operative work of infection control involving the microbiologist, infectologist or clinical microbiologist, epidemiologist and infection control nurses (ICNs) in regular discussions of the infection control situation throughout the hospital.

The number of infection control nurses is the most important factor in achieving effective control. It is recommended that there be one ICN per 200–250 beds, but at least two ICNs in small hospitals (up to 300 beds).

Documents on infection control

Documentation of infection control is essential to make it systematic and controllable. It allows the system to be monitored across time, and for intra-hospital and inter-hospital comparisons to be made.

There are three types of documentation:

- standards
- protocols
- guidelines.

Producers of documents are either:

- internal – published locally by the ICC of the hospital, or
- external – produced by the health authorities or professional institutes.

In medicine, *standards* are issued by health authorities and organizations and are the core documents on infection control. They regulate the 'structure' and/or the 'process' components of health care with the aim of ensuring that good and appropriate structures and processes can ensure appropriate outcomes (see Figure 7.1). The principle of standards is *'all or nothing'*, meaning that the specified conditions should satisfy the requirements of standards. Following the standards should guarantee safe procedures. A common example is the sterilization process. Acceptance of standards may be compulsory or optional, depending on the health policy of the country concerned.

The geographical extent of standards may be:

- international
- national.

International standards produced by international organizations such as WHO or the European Union may be optional for individual countries, but the aim is harmonization and standardization of health care among different countries, making comparisons possible (see Annexe 2).

National standards, issued by the health authorities of individual countries, are valid within the borders of that country. Standards of different countries regulating the same issue can differ, sometimes inexplicably. The ICC of a hospital must be familiar with its national standards, and adhere to them.

Protocols regulate specific 'processes' step by step, for example the insertion of sterile devices, surgical hand-washing, etc. They may be issued by professional organizations or by the local ICC.

The purposes of protocols are to:

- fill the gap if there are no existing standards for a particular process
- give guidance when a process may be carried out in alternative ways
- minimize the cost, while keeping the efficacy at the same level or higher.

Guidelines are usually produced by professional organizations. Their observance is optional as they have only the force of a recommendation. The local ICC may adopt existing guidelines, or produce their own according to the local circumstances in the absence of professional recommendations.

The local documentation of infection control in hospital is usually the *Infection Control Manual (ICM)*. Its various parts regulate the whole process of infection control in the hospital by specifying exactly: *who should do ..., what should be done ..., when it should be done ..., how it should be done ....* Regular updating by the ICC is recommended to maintain quality control. Standards, protocols and guidelines are the essential parts of an ICM.

Measures of hospital-acquired infection

The best way to characterize the outcomes of health care is by objective evaluation. Two methods are accepted nowadays:

- quantitative
- qualitative.

The *quantitative analysis* of health care uses mathematical terms to describe the outcome and magnitude of HAI in terms of rates, ratios and proportions. It uses highly sophisticated statistical analyses about the causal inferences, and determinants of HAI and the outcome. Quantitative analysis needs advanced professional epidemiological and statistical knowledge. The types of data and statistical operations are the same as those required for other statistical and epidemiological research:

- continuous – for example, age, duration of operation
- discrete:
  - ordinal – for example, severity of disease (mild, intermediate, severe, lethal)
  - nominal – gender, presence or absence of risk factor.

In epidemiology there are three types of measures used to describe the frequency of occurrence of a health event: ratios, proportions and rates. In everyday English the word 'rate' has more than one meaning and it is a common mistake to confuse it with 'proportion' and to use it as a synonym for 'ratio' (Elandt-Johnson, 1975).

Ratio (R) is the result of dividing one quantity by another (with the same or different units), $R = a/b$, for example the sex ratio of male to female (male/female) (Elandt-Johnson, 1975). It has bounds of zero and infinity, and the unit of ratio depends on the units of the component quantities; if the units are the same for both then the measure has no units (i.e. it is expressed as a pure number).

Proportion (*p*) is a type of ratio in which the numerator is included in the denominator; $p = a/a+b$. This strict mathematical connection between the numerator and the denominator distinguishes the proportion from other measures. Every proportion is a ratio, but not every ratio is a proportion. Proportion is unitless because the numerator and the denominator have the same dimension, and the bounds are zero and one. The proportion is often called a fraction. It is the estimation of probability (*p*) of any event (Elandt-Johnson, 1975). We speak of disease frequency (*f*) if this probability is applied to a population, and the same probability is called risk (*r*) if it is applied to an individual.

Risk is defined as the probability or expected frequency of the occurrence of a harmful event. The word originates from the French: *risqué* – and from the Italian *rischia*, *risico* or *risco* = hazard, peril, – danger (Churchill's, 1989, p. 1656). A population at risk consists of those individuals who are in danger of developing a health hazard. Exposure to danger is a necessary requirement of being at risk. The word 'exposure' originates from the French: ex + *poser* = to put, to place from Latin *positus* past participle of *ponere* to place, to put (Churchill's, 1989, p. 663).

Exposure may have different attributes:

- dose of exposure – such as an infectious dose
- duration of exposure:
  - at one point in time – surgical intervention lasting for a short time
  - repeated exposure – insertion of intravenous catheters at different sites
  - continuous exposure – for example, a urinary catheter being inserted permanently.

Rate can be defined as a measure of change in one quantity (called dependent) per unit of another quantity (called independent) on which the dependent quantity depends (Elandt-Johnson, 1975). If the independent quantity is *time*, it describes a continuous process in time – the *average velocity* or speed of a process.

Depending on the attributes, two main categories of disease frequency are used:

- incidence measures
- prevalence measures.

Incidence uses the new cases occurring in the population at risk within a defined time interval, or at a point in time. Incidence estimates the risk of the development of a health event. It comes from Latin *incidentia* (from *incidere* = to happen, befall, from *in* = in, into + *cadere* = to fall) meaning happening, occurrence (Churchill's, 1989, p. 928). Proportions and rates are used for its mathematical expression.

Two types of incidence are distinguished:

- cumulative incidence
- incidence density.

Cumulative incidence (CI) – estimates the *risk* within a defined time interval (week, month or year) expressed as a proportion. It is called cumulative because the events occurring throughout the time interval are added together cumulatively, producing the total number of cases by the end of the time interval.

The general formula is:

$$\frac{\textit{Total number of people contracting the new health event during the time interval}}{\textit{Total number of population at risk in the same time interval}}$$

The critical point is the calculation of the numerator and denominator, i.e. including all the people subject to the health event, and defining the total number of population at risk. Individuals with a new health event should be counted only once in the numerator – cases of reactivation are omitted. Individuals are counted in the denominator as many times as they enter the population at risk during the observation period; if they remain at risk during the whole of the observation period without leaving, then they are counted only once.

For HAI two general estimates of cumulative incidence are used: the 'overall nosocomial infection risk' and the 'nosocomial infection risk':

Overall nosocomial infection risk is calculated as:

$$\frac{\textit{Total number of all types of new nosocomial infections during the time interval}}{\textit{Total number of discharges within the same time interval}}$$

This is wrongly called the incidence rate of HAI by many authors, even though the characteristics of 'rate' are not involved in this measure (Martone et al., 1991). It estimates the *overall* risk because it takes into account the possibility that one person may acquire more than one HAI during one hospital stay, for example pneumonia and a wound infection. We have to remember that the term 'nosocomial infection' is equivalent to 'hospital-acquired infection' in defining the *place* of acquisition of infection or the *hospital-dependence* of its development. If a patient develops a urinary tract infection he or she is still at risk of developing pneumonia, or acquiring other infections. 'Overall nosocomial risk' shows the average number of all the infections acquired per unit of discharged patients during the chosen time interval. This measure is not a true proportion but has the characteristic of a 'ratio' because the numerator and denominator do not follow the rules of proportion exactly, i.e. patients with two or more HAIs will be counted twice or more in the numerator. This measure can be expressed per 100 or per 1000 discharges, and is frequently used in publications because of its ease of calculation. A Unit [new nosocomial infections per unit of discharge] is defined for the duration of observation. It is mistake to express the measure as a percentage if the multiplier is equal to 100 because it is not a proportion.

Nosocomial infection risk:

$$\frac{\textit{Total number of patients acquiring a new specified infection during the time interval}}{\textit{Total number of population at risk of the specified infection in the same time interval}}$$

In some medical papers it is called – again wrongly – attack rate (Martone et al., 1991). It is in fact a true proportion, expressing the risk of acquiring a *specific* infection. We use it for outbreaks or for routine surveillance of a specific type of HAI, regardless of the outbreak situation. For convenience and standard comparison it can also be multiplied by 100 or 1000, expressing the number of infected patients per 100 or 1000 of the population at risk. If the multiplier is 100 then it is expressed as a percentage. However, we have to remember that the bounds of probability are always between zero and one. Thus it is advisable not to use any multiplier.

The measure 'nosocomial infection risk' is used for two purposes:

- first, when the population at risk is equal the total number of discharges, for example new urinary tract infected patients per 100 discharges per month. A Unit [newly infected patients per number of discharges] is defined for the time of observation
- second, for procedure-dependent HAI when the population at risk consists only of those who undergo the procedure; for example, the number of surgical wound infections per 100 or 1000 operations per time interval. A patient can be operated on several times at different sites, and be at risk of developing a surgical wound infection each time an operation is performed. If the patient is not operated on he or she is

not at risk of developing a surgical wound infection. This is the reason why the 'overall nosocomial risk' (counting both procedure-dependent and procedure non-dependent infections) is always biased, because the chance of acquiring all types of HAI is not the same for every discharged patient. Procedures will differ between wards and between hospitals, leading to misinterpretation when we compare them using only the overall nosocomial risk.

It is confusing if the 'nosocomial infection risk' is used instead of 'overall nosocomial risk' to estimate the overall magnitude of nosocomial infections, counting only the number of infected patients regardless of the number of nosocomial infections in each infected case. This can be applied only if each nosocomially infected patient acquires only *one* infection during his/her stay in hospital; if not, this measure underestimates the overall occurrence of nosocomial infections. This is the case in intensive care units, where patients are likely to acquire more than one nosocomial infection (see Figure 7.4). The bigger the gap between the values of the overall nosocomial infection risk and the nosocomial infection risk, the more likely it is that a patient will acquire more than one infection, on average. It is advisable to distinguish between the number of patients who acquire only one infection and those who acquire more than one.

It is also advisable to stratify the patients with nosocomial infections according to the number of different infections and estimate the risk for each stratum, i.e. estimating the risk of acquiring one, two, three, etc. infections per individual patient.

The main disadvantage of all cumulative incidence measures in routine surveillance is that the time interval is chosen arbitrarily. A month is the norm for routine surveillance of HAIs, but patients do not spend equal amounts of time at risk of acquiring HAI, and usually less than one month because the average bed occupancy in hospitals is normally less than one month. Additionally, average bed occupancy may differ between services and hospitals. Despite this, one month is the conventional period for routine HAI surveillance. This problem is avoided in an outbreak situation, when the follow-up of patients is quite precise. Furthermore, the cumulative incidence may be biased because the numerator is not always included in the denominator when the acquisition of the HAI and the time of discharge do not occur within the same time interval. For example, the patient acquires the infection in April and is counted in the denominator but is discharged in another time interval – perhaps in May or later. The

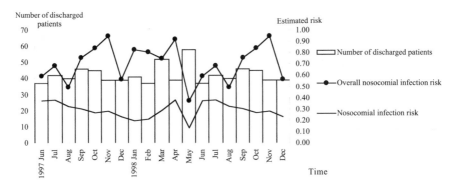

Figure 7.4. Frequency of nosocomial infections at the Intensive Care Unit of hospital 'A', Hungary, between June 1997 and December 1998.

population of a hospital is dynamic, i.e. patients admitted to the hospital enter the general risk of acquiring HAI and remain at risk during their stay in hospital. By convention the number of discharges is used in the denominator because the patients cease to be at risk of HAI after discharge. In the number of discharges we count both those who leave the hospital alive and those who die in hospital. If the patient is transferred to another hospital it counts as another admission at the receiving hospital, because the risk must be estimated for each hospital separately.

Example

In a hospital surgery unit, 127 patients were discharged alive and three patients died in the month of interest. Among 120 patients who had undergone an operation 10 patients acquired hospital infection: one patient had only surgical wound infection (SWI), three patients had SWI and pneumonia, four patients had developed SWI and urinary tract infection, and two patients had only central venous catheter (CVC) associated bloodstream infection. Among non-operated patients one CVC-associated infection occurred. The total number of patients who had CVC was five among the non-operated and 40 patients among the operated. Twenty of the patients had a urinary catheter. All patients with urinary tract infections except one in the operated group had had a urinary tract catheter.

- *Overall nosocomial infection risk*: epidemiologically it would be incorrect if we were to count all types of HAI (eight surgical wound infections, three cases of pneumonia, four urinary tract infections, and three CVC-associated infections) in the numerator (total of 18 infections), dividing by the total of 130 discharges – giving $18/130 = 0.14$ – because only 120 (92.30%) patients are at risk of SWI and only 45 (34.61%) were at risk of CVC-associated bloodstream infection. It is not advisable to report this measure.

- *Nosocomial infection risk*: 11 patients developed 18 infections altogether, so it would also be incorrect to estimate the risk counting only the infected patients (especially those who developed more than one infection) once in the numerator ($11/130$) ignoring the possibility of developing multiple infections. This measure should be avoided in this case.
- *Risk of surgical wound infection*: $8/120 = 0.666$ or 6.6 SWIs per 100 operations.
- *Risk of pneumonia*: $3/130 = 0.023$ or 2.3 cases of pneumonia per 100 discharged patients.
- *Risk of urinary tract infection*: $4/130 = 0.031$ or 3.1 urinary tract infections per 100 discharged patients.
- *Catheter-associated urinary tract infection*: $3/20 = 0.150$ or 15 urinary tract infections per 100 urinary tract catheterized patients.
- *Risk of catheter-associated bloodstream infection*: $3/45 = 0.666$ or 6.6 CVC-associated infections per 100 CVC patients.

The reader may ask whether the risk measures were appropriate or not, as shown in Figure 7.4. As mentioned above, Figure 7.4 illustrates the inappropriateness of 'nosocomial infection risk' counting only infected patients if they develop more than one infection. If all, or almost all, discharged patients have a risk of developing every possible infection (for example, in intensive care units) then overall nosocomial infection risk may be reported, but it is strongly advised to report specific incidence measures.

Precise measurement of the time is important when the risk depends on the time spent subject to the 'exposed to risk factor', which needs an additional measure called the 'incidence density'.

Incidence density (I_D) is a measure of rate, and takes into account the time of being at risk of developing a health event.

The general formula is:

$$\frac{\textit{Total number of people contracting the new health event}}{\textit{Sum of the time that each person is at risk, from among the population at risk}}$$

The relevant time unit must be specified, i.e. day, week, month or year [cases per person-day, or person-week or person-months, person-years]. In hospitals the risk is expressed in 'patient-days'. This summary measure expresses how many cases occur on average per unit time at risk. It is not a true risk measure, even if the time at risk is used for the calculation, because the total number of the population is not used directly, only the sum of the time at risk for each individual. For example, two patients each spending ten days in hospital gives a total of 20 patient-days, while one patient spending 20 days in hospital also gives 20 patient-days. For standard comparison purposes the incidence density is multiplied by 100 or 1000, obtaining the number of cases per 100 or 1000 times unit at risk. For HAI, 100 or 1000 patient-days is accepted for estimations.

Overall nosocomial incidence rate:

$$\frac{\textit{Total number of all types of new nosocomial infections}}{\textit{Sum of the time that each person is at risk (patient-days) from among the population at risk}}$$

This measure used to be called the 'incidence density' of HAI, which seems correct; however, 'rate' is more appropriate if we accept the definitions above (Elandt-Johnson, 1975). Incidence rate is usually restricted to the first event – in this case the first nosocomial infection. The time at risk runs from the first day of being at risk until the acquisition of HAI (or until discharge if the patient does not acquire HAI during hospitalization). Technically the calculation of incidence density is rather difficult because the data on being at risk has to be obtained individually, which needs a lot of time if the population at risk is large. Time at risk is not uniform for each type of HAI and may not be equal to patient-days. For procedure-dependent infections it starts at the beginning of the procedure and lasts until the end of the procedure (for example, catheter-associated urinary tract infections). But, for example, the risk of wound infection lasts from the time of the operation until the wound has totally healed, which usually occurs after discharge, but may occur before. Thus, this measure may not accurately estimate the time-dependent risk for all types of HAI using patient-days uniformly.

Nosocomial incidence rate:

$$\frac{\textit{Total number of a specific type of new nosocomial infection}}{\textit{Sum of the time that each person is at risk (patient-days) from among the population at risk}}$$

This measure is restricted to only one specific type of infection at a time, and is calculated separately for different types of infection. Accordingly different subtypes can be derived from the general formula, which is quite common in the case of device-associated infections, taking into account the exposure time with the inserted device:

- pneumonia associated with intubation or mechanical ventilation
- urinary tract infection due to indwelling catheters
- bloodstream infections associated with intravascular catheters.

Estimating of the risk of HAI has two purposes:

- estimating the occurrence of an infection in the hospital population, i.e. the expected level (endemic);
- individual risk assessment, i.e. estimating the risk of developing a HAI for each individual patient in the presence of risk factors (age, gender, underlying diseases, ASA score, APECHE score, immunosuppression, etc.) by stratified or multivariable methods.

Prevalence is the second type of disease frequency. It is the sum of *all* cases, i.e. new cases developed during the survey plus old cases who had developed the health event before the survey but which still exists at the time of the survey. Two types of prevalence measure are used:

- period prevalence – where the defined time is an interval (e.g. a week)
- point prevalence – where the defined time is one point in time, usually a day.

As the prevalence includes both new and old cases, its magnitude depends on the incidence, i.e. on the risk and on the duration of the health event. Mathematically there is an association between incidence and prevalence:

Prevalence = incidence × average duration of health event

Prevalence shows the actual number of infected patients and infections that exist at a point or during a period of time, which is a basic measure for the calculation of cost. While the incidence measures reflect the risk of infection and achievements of preventive efforts, the prevalence measures are affected by both the incidence and the ability to cure the infectious disease. Prevalence can be high with low incidence if the average duration of the infection is long, and vice versa with short average duration if the incidence is high with a similar distribution in time (in a highly endemic area).

In hospitals, point prevalence is mainly used to collect data on a particular day. This is easy to conduct and is useful for rapid screening of the epidemiological situation. Two types of prevalence measure are used: prevalence of infections and prevalence of infected patients.

Prevalence of infections

$$\frac{\textit{Total number of all types of active nosocomial infections}}{\textit{Total number of patients present at the time of survey}}$$

This measure is called – again wrongly – the 'prevalence rate'. In fact, it is a ratio, and the unit of this measure is: [infections per patient]. It shows how many infections occur on average per patient during the survey period or at one point in time. It can also be multiplied by 100 or by 1000. Percentage must not be used. Some authors have suggested that both cured and active infections be included owing to the difficulty of defining the end of the infectious process. However, the essence of point or period prevalence is to measure *only* those cases that actually have the health event of interest. Including cured cases will distort the prevalence measure by overestimating it.

Prevalence of infected patients

$$\frac{\textit{Total number patients having at least one type of active nosocomial infection}}{\textit{Total number of patients present at the time of survey}}$$

This measure underestimates the real prevalence, especially if patients develop more than one HAI. The more infections that occur on average per patient, the bigger the underestimation. This measure should therefore not be used alone, but only together with the measure of 'prevalence of infections'.

Qualitative research and analysis is the second widely used method that helps to formulate preliminary questions for quantitative research or can be used at the stage of quantitative analysis of data (Mays and Pope, 1995; Pope and Mays, 1995). Both quantitative and qualitative methods are used equally in the evaluation of infection control methods, depending on the exact purpose of the epidemiological study. In cases where the determinants or risk factors of HAI cannot be characterized quantitatively, qualitative analysis helps to explain the outcome by discovering 'what is behind the figures' (Baum, 1995). Qualitative research helps to describe the difference in surveillance and infection control activities in different hospitals and wards, which may result in different occurrence of HAI (Garner et al., 1982). While qualitative research analyses the outcome of health care, quantitative research is looking for the *structure* and *process* components (see Figure 7.2).

The main types of qualitative research are:

- observation
- interview
- analysis of content.

Observation describes the process of health care as if examining the frames of a *movie*, looking from the beginning to the end of the specified process, searching for the critical points that influence the occurrence of HAI – for example the process of skin disinfection, or hand-washing.

Interviews are used to obtain information from persons involved in the process, asking questions about the existing possibilities or practices, or the opinion of staff on a specific issue.

Analysis of the content is deep research and analysis of all questions on the subject.

Comparison of data on HAI

Comparison is the unique feature of epidemiological analysis. Comparing populations by means of their different characteristics, those risk factors can be defined that contribute to higher morbidity and mortality. Incidence and prevalence measures characterize the magnitude of a health-related event, and additionally serve to compare different populations across time and in various places (see Figure 7.5).

In hospital epidemiology these measures are used for comparison of the occurrence of HAI between hospitals, and between the different wards within a hospital. However, their values may be affected by factors other than population characteristics, and these should be taken into account if we want to compare different hospitals:

- methodological factors:
  - definitions used
  - type of measures used
  - precision of data collection
- functioning preventive measures
- population characteristics, e.g. risk factors (susceptibility to the infection).

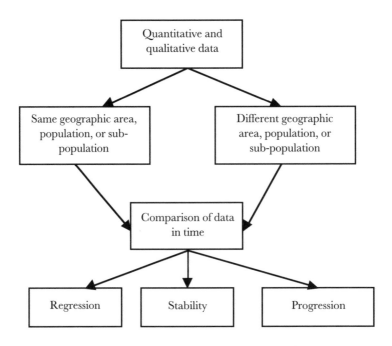

Figure 7.5. Comparison of epidemiological data.

Hospitals, and even wards, may differ in factors other than population characteristics, which makes it difficult to compare incidence and prevalence measures between hospitals, and is even meaningless where crude measures are used. Methodologies should be standardized and clearly defined for any comparison to be valid. Within a hospital it is essential to set up a comparison system when a preventive programme is implemented, because estimating the occurrence is the best way to evaluate a preventive programme.

Comparison of qualitative results is more difficult than quantitative data as their nature can be different, which makes them difficult to standardize. Standards, guidelines and protocols can be the basis for comparison of qualitative data. The extent of divergence from these documents can be determined among hospitals or wards. If these can be converted into mathematical figures the comparison is similar to quantitative data.

Data management of hospital-acquired infection

There are huge amounts of data in health care; however, infection control needs only relevant data that contain information useful in discovering possible ways of influencing the occurrence of HAI. 'Information is that intangible something which leads to enlightenment through communication; the term is linked closely with knowledge. More precisely, information is defined as the "reduction of uncertainty"' (Wilson, 1995, p. 2). Selecting relevant data and converting them into information is important to save both time and the resources of infection control. *Information is power.*

Valid data management is the basis of effective quantitative and qualitative evaluation of infection control. Data stored in hospital documentation serve mainly for the historical recall of all events of health care. They are used for legal cases, for research and for statistical purposes. It is important to understand – even if it appears to be trivial – the essentials of data collection and the documentation systems of health care in hospitals, as they have different functions.

Data have different purposes, and are recorded, stored and collected in different ways according to the:

- duration of the data collection – surveillance and surveys
- unity of the data – data for each individual patient, and aggregated
- source of data – case history or complementary documents
- technique of recording and storage – paper and computer records.

Two main methods of data collection are used in public health, which also apply to HAI (Thacker and Berkelman, 1988):

- epidemiological surveillance
- surveys.

'Surveillance, when applied to a disease means the continued watchfulness over the distribution and trends of incidence through the systematic collection, consolidation and evaluation of morbidity and mortality reports and other relevant data. Intrinsic in the concept is the regular dissemination of the basic data and interpretations to all who have contributed and to all others who need to know' (Langmuir, 1963). This definition clearly identifies the four consecutive phases of surveillance: data collection, data analysis, interpretation and dissemination of the results, and emphasizes the systematic and ongoing nature of surveillance.

The meaning of 'surveillance' originates in French: from *sur* = on, over + *veiller* = to watch + *ance* means keeping watch (Churchill's, 1989, p. 1826). This word is used if somebody is watched permanently by the police. As an epidemiological method, surveillance was first introduced in the 1960s at the Centers for Disease Control (CDC), Atlanta, GA (Langmuir, 1963; 1967).

Surveillance is an ongoing flow of information about the function of the system being investigated. Its duration may be several months or years, or even an indefinite time, until it is needed. It is widely used in the infection control of HAI, where surveillance may start with the collection of data from case histories (see Figure 7.6).

Surveillance of HAI was first used by Ignacz Semmelweis in 1846–47, although it was not then called surveillance (Semmelweis, 1861). In the twentieth century, with the resurgence of the problem of HAI, various methods of surveillance were evaluated (Eickhoff et al., 1969).

With the development of epidemiology, internal evaluation of surveillance has been developed, with different criteria to ensure that it is functioning so as to meet the system's objectives (Klaucke et al., 1988; Thacket et al. 1988).

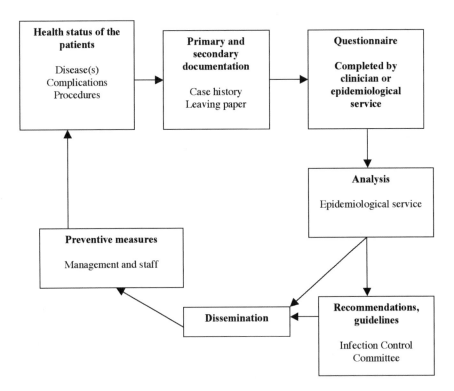

Figure 7.6. Connection of surveillance of HAI with prevention.

Uses of surveillance:

- Monitoring:
  - to detect changes in the frequency and distribution of health events
  - for observation of trends (expected level) and/or patterns in health events
  - to detect any changes in hosts and/or infectious agents
  - to follow up any changes in health practice that may influence the outcome.
- Prevention:
  - to extend our knowledge about the focuses of health events, about the transmission of infectious agents and to determine priorities if prevention is quite achievable
  - for evaluation of the efficacy of existing preventive measures
  - for the design of new methods of prevention.
- Public health research:
  - formulation of hypotheses about the health event under surveillance.

Types of surveillance according to the method of collecting or reporting the data:

- passive or routine reporting – data collected and reported by a non-epidemiologist, usually clinical or other staff;
- active – data collected by a trained epidemiologist, infection control nurses or other epidemiological assistants;
- sentinel – specially trained clinicians or other non-epidemiologist staff collect the data on a voluntary basis.

In Hungary, passive compulsory ward notification surveillance of 12 types of HAI (postoperative wound infections, oedema malignum, complications after birth, sepsis, pneumonia, interstitial pneumonia, varicella, enteritis-enterocolitis, pyoderma-impetigo-pemphigoid, urinary tract infections, abscess after injection, and thrombophlebitis) applied between 1973 and 1991. This reporting system had serious drawbacks:

- no standard definitions were adopted
- risk was not properly estimated because the denominator, i.e. the true population at risk, was not determined; instead it was taken to be only the absolute cases published by the National Institute for Public Health, Budapest.

For rough international comparison, I have made an attempt to convert raw data estimating the overall crude nosocomial infection risk, using the reported cases and the number of all discharged patients (obtained from the reports of the National Institute for Statistics, Budapest) with due regard to the fact that the population at risk might not be the same where the reported cases arose (see Figure.7.7).

Cases per 100 discharged patients

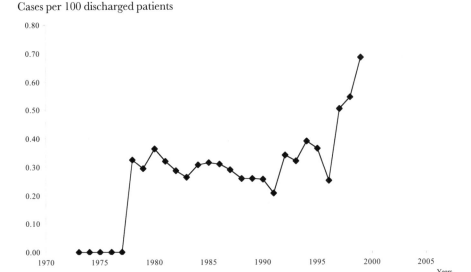

Figure 7.7. Estimated overall risk of nosocomial infections according to reported cases throughout Hungary between 1973 and 1999.

It is difficult to evaluate this reporting system because of lack of parallel use of reference surveillance. However, there is a feeling that there was some under-reporting. In 1991 this passive reporting system became optional, but the same unbelievably low trends for HAI are still reported in Hungary (see Figure 7.7).

Difference occurs in detection precision between passive and active surveillance with lower reporting in passive data provision (Vogt et al., 1983). This can explain, logically, that data on the occurrence of HAI collected passively in Hungary are much lower than that found in the active surveillance in the USA; in other countries even the population and other determinants are different (Howard et al., 1964; Ayliffe et al., 1977; Haley et al., 1985b; Moro et al., 1986; Mertens et al., 1987; Glenister et al., 1992a, 1992b).

A much higher occurrence of HAI was detected in the USA with active surveillance in the Study of the Efficacy of Nosocomial Infection Control (SENIC) programme (Haley et al., 1985b).

According to the size of the hospital population involved in the surveillance, it can be:

*   general (or hospital-wide)
*   targeted (or selected).

In *hospital-wide surveillance*, data are collected on all infections throughout the whole hospital population, which is time consuming because of the large amount of data to be collected and analysed. Hospital-wide surveillance is not recommended except for a short time (a maximum of six months) to obtain baseline data and to identify the critical wards and populations.

Target surveillance takes less time, and more informative data can be collected per unit of time, with easier and more detailed statistical analysis, which is more feasible and useful. The golden rule in hospitals is: '*Extensive surveillance – no results, targeted surveillance – good results.*' The infection control nurse or assistant should not spend more than 50% of the working day on surveillance; the remaining time should be devoted to other activities – especially to preventive interventions.

Usually the name of the surveillance refers to the starting point. The relative efficacy of eight types of active surveillance has been evaluated for HAI (Glenister et al., 1992b):

*   laboratory-based ward surveillance (LBWS) – beginning with the reporting of laboratory data and continuing on the wards by review of medical histories
*   laboratory-based telephone surveillance (LBTS) – reporting laboratory data and exchanging information by telephone
*   ward liaison surveillance (WLS) – starts in the wards by collecting information from medical histories
*   laboratory-based ward liaison surveillance (LBWLS) – a combination of LBWS and WLS methods
*   risk factor surveillance (RFS) – selecting patients by defined risk factors in the wards
*   temperature chart surveillance (TPS) – selecting patients by reviewing temperature charts
*   treatment chart surveillance (TXS) – selecting patients receiving antibiotics by reviewing treatment charts

- temperature and treatment chart surveillance (TPXS) – a combination of the TPS and TXS methods.

A *survey* is non-continuous data collection, within a specific time frame, i.e. it has defined start and end points. It may be a point in time (usually a day) or a limited period lasting from some days to weeks, or rarely some months. A survey may be *single* – collecting data only once, or *repeated* when collection of the same data is carried out periodically (see Figure 7.8). Surveys usually take less time to collect data; however, there are always gaps in data collection, i.e. information about events occurring between consecutive surveys will be missing (see Figure 7.8). If the risk of HAI is distributed about equally among consecutive time intervals, repeated surveys will reveal the same risk. A repeated survey is appropriate if data collection is followed by the implementation of preventive measures to ensure their effectiveness. Surveys are also used for epidemiological research if more data are required than can be collected by routine surveillance.

The survey method was used to evaluate the combined and independent effects of the *surveillance* and *control activities* (preventive actions) in the SENIC (Study of the Efficacy of Nosocomial Infection Control) project using the retrospective chart review of 339 044 patients in 3599 hospitals throughout the USA by comparing the occurrence of nosocomial urinary tract infection, surgical wound infection, pneumonia and bacteremia in 1970 and 1975–76 (Haley et al., 1985b). Series of papers were published throughout the study design and analysis period informing the public about the progress of the project (Haley et al. 1980a; Haley et al., 1980b; Haley et al., 1980c; Haley et al., 1980d; Hooton et al., 1980; Whaley et al., 1980; Quade et al., 1980a; Quade et al., 1980b; Haley et al., 1981a; Haley et al., 1981b; Haley et al., 1985a, 1985b, 1985c; Haley 1981; 1985). The SENIC

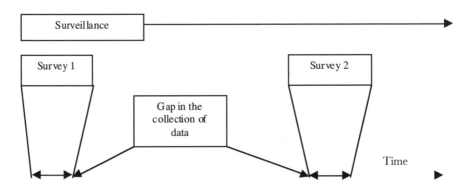

Figure 7.8. Collection of data by surveillance and surveys.

programme has been the most imposing event in the history of hospital epidemiology since the work of Semmelweis in 1847–48. Interestingly, no one was able to repeat the SENIC study, even in the USA. It was found that the occurrence of HAI decreased by 32% on average in those hospitals where programmes were implemented while the occurrence increased by 18% in those where no effective (or no) programmes were established (Haley et al., 1985c). However, it must be emphasized that surveillance alone does not prevent HAI. It becomes effective and useful if the information obtained by surveillance promotes effective preventive measures. Effectiveness of surveillance should not be confused with effectiveness of prevention: 'The concept, however, does not encompass direct responsibility for control activities' (Langmuir, 1963). Preventive actions are effective without surveillance, but most of the results will be invisible. Surveillance alone will never be effective without preventive measures, although it may have an indirect effect psychologically, influencing those who are take part in the implementation and use of preventive measures.

It is a unique feature of epidemiology to count individual cases of health events, to classify them into sub-populations according to different characteristics, and then to compare the frequencies of health events in those sub-populations to identify high-risk populations. This needs collection of data of different extents to achieve the epidemiological purpose. According to the extent of data collected they can be:

- individual;
- aggregated.

Individual data consist of variables that are characteristic of each individual. Questionnaires are used to collect data on individuals from different available data sources. This makes data collection a standardized procedure, it is easier, processing is quicker and the recall of the variables is more precise.

Aggregated data are the result of statistical summarization of individual or of any other types of data. They may come from a primary source, when the aggregated data are produced directly by a non-epidemiologist and the epidemiologist chooses the appropriate data from the data set. They can also be collected by an epidemiologist, using only relevant variables from the individual data.

It is most important that loss of data during collection or analysis should be minimized to less than 10%, or the study will lose its precision. This affects both the surveillance and survey methods, and applies regardless of individual or aggregated data (see Figure 7.9).

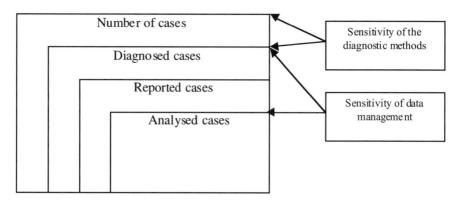

Figure 7.9. Loss of data during an epidemiological study.

There is no compensatory method in the statistical analysis if the missed data cannot be retrieved later by repeating the collection process. This is illustrated in Table 7.1, where the proportion of missed information is calculated.

Table 7.1. Results of the post-discharge surveillance of postoperative wound infections in two surgical departments at hospital 'A', Hungary, between 2 January 1995 and 31 March 1995.

Documentation of wound on control sheet	Discharged patients	
	Number	**Percentage**
Control sheet was missing from the case history	238	70.2
No wound infection found (documented)	64	18.9
No data about the wound infection on the control sheet	31	9.1
Wound infection documented	6	1.8
Total	**339**	**100.0**

The higher the proportion of real cases to analysed cases, the better the whole detection system. The detection system should be checked internally by evaluating the diagnostic procedures, the reporting system and the analysis.

The *data source* is the point at which collection of the data begins. In hospitals it may be in the form of:

- medical records
- background documents (i.e. other than medical records).

The *medical record* of each individual patient is the primary document. The health condition of the patient and all medical actions carried out on the patient as the subject of health care are recorded in this document. Clinical staff are responsible for the correctness of medical records and should validate the entries with their signature.

The primary functions of medical records are to:

- recall all the information about each patient for future use if readmission occurs
- provide evidence in case of any legal dispute over the diagnosis and treatment.

In medico-legal cases the experts rely mainly on this document, and the court will blame the hospital if any important information is missing from the medical record. The principle is: 'If anything is not documented then it has not been done'. It should be emphasized that the normal physiological condition of the patient should also be recorded, because the absence of such data may expose staff to accusations of negligence.

The secondary functions of medical records are to provide:

- information for research
- individual data for practical statistics.

Background documents should record all the actions that are performed to promote health care, apart from the primary health care of patients. They do not form part of the medical records. Their function is to describe the whole structure and process in a hospital, regardless of individual patients. They are recorded by specialist personnel who are in charge of specific functions, for example documents on laundry control, catering, drug utility, disinfectants, etc. Their function is mainly operational or statistical, but there may be legal implications as well. For infection control, the main background documents are:

- records of pharmacy and other supplies – use of disinfectants, antibiotics
- laboratory data – antibiotic resistance map of the hospital
- data from other diagnostic centres – annual statistics
- recording ward rounds and visits to patients – information for qualitative analysis
- finance – cost of infection control and other activities.

The format of data storage may be:

- paper records
- computer records.

Paper recording stores data as they were originally written – either manually or typed. This format is compulsory for medico-legal cases, and medical records should always be stored in this way.

Advantages of paper records:

- data remain in the original format unless they are manipulated later
- flexibility, i.e. the format of the sheets can be changed easily according to the purpose and type of the data
- validation by original signature.

Disadvantages of paper records:

- records need a large amount of storage space, especially in big hospitals
- not convenient for a quick search through large amounts of data
- special preparation required for statistical analysis
- not always available at the time of data collection
- there are no back-up copies, so records may be lost
- data may be incomplete – many people are involved in producing the documentation
- the health care provided and the record may differ, i.e. data may not be valid
- only routine data are recorded – they are not research oriented.

Computer recorded data are stored in a format that uses analogue or digital technology. Data are usually entered manually into the computer from other primary sources, thus they become secondary sources. Computer recording needs an appropriate hardware system (server, computers, printers, monitors, etc.) with appropriate software programs, all of which increase the cost of health care, but it is impossible to imagine modern health care and infection control without computerization. In hospitals two main computer systems are usually operating at the same time:

- the main hospital network
- independent computer stations with their own software programs.

The *hospital network system* has many advantages, one of the most important of which is to save time in everyday operational work.

Advantages of the network:

- large amounts of data can be stored, which many people can access at the same time via local terminals, thus increasing the database
- follow-up and identification of patients if they move from one department to another
- storing laboratory data – both clinical and microbiological
- control of the supply and use of drugs in different departments
- improved communication with staff by sending messages via an e-mail system
- educational purposes
- transferring protocols and documents
- access to the Internet, intranet or other databases
- improvement of statistical analysis: quicker preparation and download of large data sets, more extended analysis
- back-up copies can be stored
- general programs can be installed on the network system.

Adverse points of the computer network:

- mistakes may occur during entry of data
- loss of data in the electronic system
- inadvertent overwriting
- crash of the system may paralyse or delay operational work
- it is easy to manipulate the original data; unauthorized personnel with professional experience of computer languages can deliberately alter the function after cracking the passwords, from outside or inside the hospital
- 'computer viruses' may destroy the data
- continuous maintenance and development are required to accommodate the ever-increasing amounts of data
- compatible computer terminals are necessary.

Independent computer stations are used if the data are confidential and user access needs to be limited. Their capacity to store data is much less than that of a central network system. These personal computer (PC) stations are also used for specialized purposes, using tailor-made software programs other than those on the network system. This is usually the case with epidemiology.

There is no one perfect software program that can do every kind of operation (text editing, data entry, statistical analysis, graphics, data export or import, etc.), thus several programs should be available to compensate for the disadvantages of different software programs. Infection control personnel are advised to consult computer specialists in the set-up of software programs. The next points – while not exhaustive – are recommended to be taken into account in designing computer systems:

- compatibility – immediate transfer, between different programs using different computer languages
- user friendliness – easy to operate
- flexibility – with many options, which the user decides
- stability of the program – safety of operation
- amount of memory needed for operation
- space needed for storage of data.

Summary

This chapter describes the organization of infection control systems in hospitals. The following points are important:

- Nosocomial infections are negative indicators of the quality of health care; they can be decreased if infection control is part of quality control.
- 'Microbiology – infectology – hospital epidemiology' is the essential triad of qualified infection control, the failure of any element of which will result in incompleteness of infection control.
- Infection control encompasses traditional hospital hygiene and epidemiology that has been developed to analyse statistically the causes and determinants of nosocomial infections.
- Different types of incidence and prevalence measures are used to estimate the occurrence of different nosocomial infections in surveys or continuous data collection, and provide different messages serving different purposes.
- It is crucial that the correct terminology in hospital epidemiology be applied to standard measures, definitions and data collection methods.
- Ratios, proportions and rates should be used in accordance with their correct meaning, as Elandt-Johnson proposed, naming and defining appropriate estimates of the risk of nosocomial infections.

- If the time interval (window period) is arbitrarily chosen (i.e. months, years, etc.) then *ratios* and *proportions* are used to estimate the risk of nosocomial infections. *Rates* are used to express the average velocity of nosocomial infections.
- Surveillance is not the same as preventive efforts, being purely an epidemiological method of data management.
- It is advisable to keep an epidemiological diary recording all the possible events influencing the occurrence of HAI.
- Computerization has increased the speed of data management and information exchange, which accelerates the process of infection control.

References

Ackerman MH (1994) The systematic inflammatory response, sepsis, and multiple organ dysfunction: new definitions for an old problem. Critical Care Nursing of Clinics of North America 6(2): 243–50.

Alvarado CJ, Stolz SM, Maki DG (1991) Nosocomial infections from contaminated endoscopes: a flawed automated endoscope washer. An investigation using molecular epidemiology. American Journal of Medicine 91(3B): 272S–280S.

Anderson RM, May RM (1991) Infectious Diseases in Humans: Dynamics and Control. Oxford: Oxford University Press.

Archer GL, Pennell E (1990) Detection of methicillin resistance in staphylococci by using DNA probe. Antimicrobial Agents and Chemotherapy 34(9): 1720–4.

Austin DJ, Anderson RM (1999) Transmission dynamics of epidemic methicillin-resistant Staphylococcus aureus and vancomycin-resistant enterococci in England and Wales. Journal of Infectious Disease 179(4): 883–91.

Ayliffe GA, Brightwell KM, Collins BJ, Lowbury EJ, Goonatilake PC, Etheridge RA (1977) Surveys of hospital infection in the Birmingham region, I: Effect of age, sex, length of stay and antibiotic use on nasal carriage of tetracycline-resistant Staphylococcus aureus and on post-operative wound infection. Journal of Hygiene (Lond) 79(2): 299–314.

Balk RA, Bone RC (1989) The septic syndrome. Definition and clinical implications. Critical Care Clinics 5(1): 1–8.

Baselski VS, Wunderink RG (1994) Bronchoscopic diagnosis of pneumonia. Clinical Microbiology Reviews 7(4): 533–58.

Baum F (1995) Researching public health: behind the qualitative–quantitative methodological debate. Social Science of Medicine 40(4): 459–68.

Beaglehole R, Bonita R, Kjellström T (1993) Basic Epidemiology. Geneva: World Health Organization.

Bethune DW, Blowers R, Parker M, Pask EA (1965) Dispersal of Staphylococcus aureus by patient and surgical staff. Lancet 27: 480–3.

Bobowick AR, Brody JA, Matthews MR, Roos R, Gajdusek DC (1973) Creutzfeldt-Jakob disease: a case-control study. American Journal of Epidemiology 98(5): 381–94.

Bone RC (1994) Sepsis and its complications: the clinical problem. Critical Care Medicine 22(7): S8–11.

Bone RC (1996) The sepsis syndrome. Definition and general approach to management. Clinical Chest Medicine 17(2): 175–81.

Brown P, Will RG, Bradley R, Asher DM, Detwiler L (2001) Bovine spongiform encephalopathy and variant Creutzfeldt-Jakob disease: background, evolution, and current concerns. Emerging Infectious Diseases 7(1): 6–14.

Bruckner DA, Colonna P, Bearson BL (1999) Nomenclature for aerobic and facultative bacteria. Clinical Infectious Disease 29(4): 713–723. [Comment: Clinical Infectious Disease (2000) 30(6): 988–9.]

Camargos PA, Guimaraes MD, Antunes CM (1988) Risk assessment for acquiring meningitis tuberculosis among children not vaccinated with BCG: a case-control study. International Journal of Epidemiology 17(1): 193–7.

Celis R, Torres A, Gatell JM, Almela M, Rodriguez-Roisin R, Agusti-Vidal A (1988) Nosocomial pneumonia. A multivariate analysis of risk and prognosis. Chest 93(2): 318–24.

Centers for Disease Control (1970) Isolation Techniques for Use in Hospitals, 1st edn. DHEW publication no. (PHS) 70–2054. Washington, DC: US Government Printing Office.

Centers for Disease Control (1975) Isolation Techniques for Use in Hospitals, 2nd edn. HHS publication no. (CDC) 80–8314. Washington, DC: US Government Printing Office.

Centers for Disease Control (1981) Guidelines for the Prevention and Control of Nosocomial Infections. Atlanta: US Department of Health and Human Services.

Centers for Disease Control (1987) Recommendations for prevention of HIV transmission in health-care settings. Morbidity and Mortality Weekly Report 36 (Suppl. 2): 1S–18S.

Centers for Disease Control (1988) Update: Universal precautions for preventing of human immunodeficiency virus, transmission of hepatitis B and other blood borne pathogens in health care settings. Morbidity and Mortality Weekly Report 37: 377–88.

Chin J (Ed) (2000) Control of Communicable Diseases Manual. Washington, DC: American Public Health Association.

Churchill's Illustrated Medical Dictionary (1989) New York, Edinburgh: Churchill Livingstone.

Coello R, Glynn JR, Gaspar C, Picazo JJ, Fereres J (1997) Risk factors for developing clinical infection with methicillin-resistant Staphylococcus aureus (MRSA) amongst hospital patients initially only colonized with MRSA. Journal of Hospital Infection 37(1): 39–46.

Cookson B, Peters B, Webster M, Phillips I, Rahman M, Noble W (1989) Staff carriage of epidemic methicillin-resistant Staphylococcus aureus. Journal of Clinical Microbiology 27(7): 1471–6. [Comment: Journal of Clinical Microbiology (1990) 28(10): 2380–1.]

Crowe MJ, Cooke EM (1998) Review of case definitions for nosocomial infection — towards a consensus. Presentation by the Nosocomial Infection Surveillance Unit (NISU) to the Hospital Infection Liaison Group, subcommittee of the Federation of Infection Societies (FIS). Journal of Hospital Infection 39(1): 3–11.

Cruse PJ, Foord R (1980) The epidemiology of wound infection. A 10-year prospective study of 62,939 wounds. Surgical Clinics of North America 60(1): 27–40.

Culver DH, Horan TC, Gaynes RP, Martone WJ, Jarvis WR, Emori TG, Banerjee SN, Edwards JR, Tolson JS, Henderson TS, et al. (1991) Surgical wound infection rates by wound class, operative procedure, and patient risk index. National Nosocomial Infections Surveillance System. American Journal of Medicine 91(3B): 152S–157S.

Daifuku R, Stamm WE (1986) Bacterial adherence to bladder uroepithelial cells in catheter-associated urinary tract infection. New England Journal of Medicine 314(19): 1208–13.

Dickinson GM, Bisno AL (1989a) Infections associated with indwelling devices: infections related to extravascular devices. Antimicrobial Agents and Chemotherapy 33(5): 602–7.

Dickinson GM, Bisno AL (1989b) Infections associated with indwelling devices: concepts of pathogenesis; infections associated with intravascular devices. Antimicrobial Agents and

Chemotherapy 33(5): 597–601. [Comment: Antimicrobial Agents and Chemotherapy (1989) 33(11): 2023.]

Donabedian (1978) The quality of medical care. Science 200(4344): 856–64.

Dorland's Illustrated Medical Dictionary (1988) Philadelphia: WB Saunders (p. 1152).

Dripps RD, Lamont A, Eckenhoff JE (1961) The role of anesthesia in surgical mortality. Journal of American Medical Association 178(3): 261–6.

Edmondson EB, Reinarz JA, Pierce AK, Sanford JP (1966) Nebulization equipment. A potential source of infection in gram-negative pneumonias. American Journal of Disease of Children 111(4): 357–60.

Eickhoff TC (1979) Epidemiology of Legionnaires' disease. Annals of Internal Medicine 90(4): 499–502.

Eickhoff TC, Brachman PW, Bennett JV, Brown JF (1969) Surveillance of nosocomial infections in community hospitals. I. Surveillance methods, effectiveness, and initial results. Journal of Infectious Disease 120(3): 305–17.

Elandt-Johnson RC (1975) Definition of rates: some remarks on their use and misuse. American Journal of Epidemiology 102(4): 267–71.

European Directorate for the Quality of Medicines (1997) European Pharmacopoeia, 3rd edn, Suppl. 2001 with revisions. Strasbourg: Council of Europe.

Fauquet CM, Pringle CR (1999) Abbreviations for vertebrate virus species names. Archives of Virology 144(9): 1865–80.

Fine PEM (1989) The BCG story: lessons from the past and implications for the future. Review of Infectious Disease 11(Suppl. 2): S353–9.

Foster WD, Hutt MSR (1960) Experimental staphylococcal infections in man. Lancet 121(2): 1373–6.

Fry DE (2000) Sepsis syndrome. American Surgery 66(2): 126–32.

Gajdusek DC, Gibbs CJ Jr, Asher DM, Brown P, Diwan A, Hoffman P, Nemo G, Rohwer R, White L (1977) Precautions in medical care of, and in handling materials from, patients with transmissible virus dementia (Creutzfeldt-Jakob disease). New England Journal of Medicine 297(23): 1253–8.

Garcia LS (1999) Classification of human parasites, vectors, and similar organisms. Clinical Infectious Diseases 29(4): 734–6.

Garfield MD, Ershler WB, Maki DG (1978) Malaria transmission by platelet concentrate transfusion. Journal of American Medical Association 240(21): 2285–6.

Garner JS (1986) CDC guideline for prevention of surgical wound infections, 1985. Supersedes guideline for prevention of surgical wound infections published in 1982. (Originally published November 1985). Revised: Infection Control 7(3): 193–200.

Garner JS (1996a) Guideline for isolation precautions in hospitals, Part I: Evolution of isolation practices, Hospital Infection Control Practices Advisory Committee. American Journal of Infection Control 24(1): 24–31.

Garner JS (1996b) Guideline for isolation precautions in hospitals. The Hospital Infection Control Practices Advisory Committee. Infection Control and Hospital Epidemiology 17(1): 53–80. [Erratum: Infection Control and Hospital Epidemiology (1996)17(4): 214.]

Garner JS, Emori TG, Haley RW (1982) Operating room practices for the control of infection in US hospitals, October 1976 to July 1977. Surgery of Gynecology and Obstetrics 155(6): 873–80.

Garner JS, Jarvis WR, Emori TG, Horan TC, Hughes JM (1988) CDC definitions for nosocomial infections, 1988. American Journal of Infection Control 16(3): 128–40. [Erratum: American Journal of Infection Control (1988) 16(4): 177.]

Garner JS, Simmons BP (1983) Guidelines for isolation precautions in hospitals. Infection Control 4(4 Suppl.): 245–325.

Gibbs CJ Jr, Gajdusek DC, Latarjet R (1978) Unusual resistance to ionizing radiation of the viruses of kuru, Creutzfeldt-Jakob disease, and scrapie. Proceedings of the National Academy of Science USA 75(12): 6268–70.

Glenister HM, Taylor LJ, Bartlett CL, Cooke EM, Mackintosh CA, Leigh DA (1992a) An 11-month incidence study of infections in wards of a district general hospital. Journal of Hospital Infection 21(4): 261–73.

Glenister HM, Taylor LJ, Cooke EM, Bartlett CLR (1992b) A Study of Surveillance Methods for Detecting Hospital Infection. London: Public Health Laboratory Service.

Glupczinsky Y, Gordts B, Melin P, Mertens R, Struelens M (1994) Guidelines for control and prevention of methicillin-resistant Staphylococcus aureus transmission in Belgian hospitals. Acta Clinica Belgica 49(2): 108–13.

Goonatilake PC (1985) Empirical and mathematical models on the relationship between patient age and nosocomial infection. International Journal of Biomedical Computing 16(3–4): 231–43.

Greene JN (1996) The microbiology of colonization, including techniques for assessing and measuring colonization. Infection Control and Hospital Epidemiology 17(2): 114–18.

Haley RW (1981) The usefulness of a conceptual model in the study of the efficacy of infection surveillance and control programs. Review of Infectious Disease 3(4): 775–80.

Haley RW (1985) Surveillance by objective: a new priority-directed approach to the control of nosocomial infections. The National Foundation for Infectious Diseases Lecture. American Journal of Infection Control 13(2): 78–89.

Haley RW, Hooton TM, Schoenfelder JR, Crossley KB, Quade D, Stanley RC, Culver DH (1980a) Effect of an infection surveillance and control program on the accuracy of retrospective chart review. American Journal of Epidemiology 111(5): 543–5.

Haley RW, Quade D, Freeman HE, Bennett JV (1980b) The SENIC Project. Study on the efficacy of nosocomial infection control (SENIC Project). Summary of study design. American Journal of Epidemiology 111(5): 472–85.

Haley RW, Schaberg DR, McClish DK, Quade D, Crossley KB, Culver DH, Morgan WM, McGowan JE Jr, Shachtman RH (1980c) The accuracy of retrospective chart review in measuring nosocomial infection rates. Results of validation studies in pilot hospitals. American Journal of Epidemiology 111(5): 516–33.

Haley RW, Schaberg DR, Von Allmen SD, McGowan JE Jr (1980d) Estimating the extra charges and prolongation of hospitalization due to nosocomial infections: a comparison of methods. Journal of Infection Disease 141(2): 248–57.

Haley RW, Culver DH, Emori TG, Hooton TM, White JW (1981a) Progress report on the evaluation of the efficacy of infection surveillance and control programs. American Journal of Medicine 70(4): 971–5.

Haley RW, Hooton TM, Culver DH, Stanley RC, Emori TG, Hardison CD, Quade D, Shachtman RH, Schaberg DR, Shah BV, Schatz GD (1981b) Nosocomial infections in US hospitals, 1975–1976: estimated frequency by selected characteristics of patients. American Journal of Medicine 70(4): 947–59.

Haley RW, Schaberg DR, Crossley KB, Von Allmen SD, McGowan JE Jr (1981c) Extra charges and prolongation of stay attributable to nosocomial infections: a prospective interhospital comparison. American Journal Medicine Jan; 70(1): 51–58.

Haley RW, Culver DH, Morgan WM, White JW, Emori TG, Hooton TM (1985a) Identifying patients at high risk of surgical wound infection. A simple multivariate index of patient susceptibility and wound contamination. American Journal of Epidemiology 121(2): 206–15.

Haley RW, Culver DH, White JW, Morgan WM, Emori TG, Munn VP, Hooton TM (1985b) The efficacy of infection surveillance and control programs in preventing nosocomial infections in US hospitals. American Journal of Epidemiology 121(2): 182–205.

Haley RW, Garner JS, Simmons BP (1985c) A new approach to the isolation of hospitalized patients with infectious diseases: alternative systems. Journal of Hospital Infection 6(2): 128–39.

Hillis A (1979) A mathematical model for the epidemiologic study of infectious diseases. International Journal of Epidemiology 8(2): 167–76.

Hooton TM, Haley RW, Culver DH (1980) A method for classifying patients according to the nosocomial infection risks associated with diagnoses and surgical procedures. American Journal of Epidemiology 111(5): 556–73.

Horan TC, Gaynes RP, Martone WJ, Jarvis WR, Emori TG (1992a) CDC definitions of nosocomial surgical site infections, 1992: a modification of CDC definitions of surgical wound infections. American Journal of Infection Control 20(5): 271–74.

Horan TC, Gaynes RP, Martone WJ, Jarvis WR, Emori TG (1992b) CDC definitions of nosocomial surgical site infections, 1992: a modification of CDC definitions of surgical wound infections. Infection Control and Hospital Epidemiology 13(10): 606–8.

Hospital Infection Society and British Society for Antimicrobial Chemotherapy (1990) Report of a combined working party: Revised guidelines for the control of epidemic methicillin-resistant Staphylococcus aureus. Journal of Hospital Infection 16(4): 351–77.

Howard JM, Barker WF Culbertson W (1964) Postoperative wound infection: the influence of ultraviolet irradiation on the operating room and of various other factors. Annals of Surgery 160 (Suppl. 2): 1–196.

Jencks SF, Dobson A (1987) Refining case-mix adjustment. The research evidence. New England Journal of Medicine 317(11): 679–86.

Johanson WG, Pierce AK, Sanford JP (1969) Changing pharyngeal bacterial flora of hospitalized patients. Emergence of gram-negative bacilli. New England Journal of Medicine 281(21): 1137–40.

Jousimies-Somer H, Summanen P (1999) Microbiology terminology update: clinically significant anaerobic gram-positive and gram-negative bacteria (excluding spirochetes). Clinical Infectious Disease 29(4): 724–7.

Kaiser AB (1986) Antimicrobial prophylaxis in surgery. New England Journal of Medicine 315(18): 1129–38.

Karzai W, Reinhart K (1998) Sepsis: definitions and diagnosis. International Journal of Clinical Practice 95(June, Suppl.): 44–8.

Keats AS (1978) The ASA classification of physical status: a recapitulation. Anesthesiology 49(4): 233–6.

Klaucke DN, Buehler JW, Thacker SB, Parrish RG, Trowbridge FL, Berkelman RL (1988) Guidelines for Evaluating Surveillance Systems. Morbidity and Mortality Weekly Report 37(No.S-5 Suppl.): 1–18.

Langmuir AD (1963) The surveillance of communicable disease of national importance. New England Journal of Medicine 268(4): 182–92.

Langmuir AD (1976) William Farr: founder of modern concepts of surveillance. International Journal of Epidemiology 5(1): 13–18.

Last JM (1995) A Dictionary of Epidemiology, 3rd edn. New York, Oxford: Oxford University Press.

Levine WC, Smart JF, Archer DL, Bean NH, Tauxe RV (1991) Foodborne disease outbreaks in nursing homes, 1975 through 1987. Journal of American Medical Association 266(15): 2105–9.

Lynch P, Cummings MJ, Roberts PL, Herriott MJ, Yates B, Stamm WE (1990) Implementing and evaluating a system of generic infection precautions: body substance isolation. American Journal of Infection Control 18(1): 1–12.

Lynch P, Jackson MM, Cummings MJ, Stamm WE (1987) Rethinking the role of isolation practices in the prevention of nosocomial infections. Annals of Internal Medicine 107(2): 243–6.

Maki DG, Botticelli JT, LeRoy ML, Thielke TS (1987) Prospective study of replacing administration sets for intravenous therapy at 48- vs 72-hour intervals. 72 hours is safe and cost-effective. Journal of American Medical Association 258(13): 1777–81.

Maki DG, Rhame FS, Mackel DC, Bennett JV (1976) Nationwide epidemic of septicemia caused by contaminated intravenous products, I: Epidemiologic and clinical features. American Journal of Medicine 60(4): 471–85.

Mangram AJ, Horan TC, Pearson ML, Silver LC, Jarvis WR (1999a) Guideline for prevention of surgical site infection, 1999. Hospital Infection Control Practices Advisory Committee. Infection Control and Hospital Epidemiology 20(4): 250–78; quiz 279–80. [Comment: Infection Control and Hospital Epidemiology (1999) 20(4): 231–2.]

Mangram AJ, Horan TC, Pearson ML, Silver LC, Jarvis WR (1999b) Guideline for Prevention of Surgical Site Infection, 1999. Centers for Disease Control and Prevention (CDC) Hospital Infection Control Practices Advisory Committee. American Journal of Infection Control 27(2): 97–132; quiz 133–4; discussion.

Martone WJ, Gaynes RP, Horan TC, Emori TG, Jarvis WR, Bennett ME, Culver DH, Banerjee SN, Edwards JR, Henderson TS, Tolson JS, Reid CR (1991) Report from the CDC: Nosocomial Infection Rates for Interhospital Comparison: Limitations and Possible Solutions. Infection Control and Hospital Epidemiology 12(10): 609–21.

Maslow J, Mulligan ME (1996) Epidemiologic typing systems. Infection Control and Hospital Epidemiology 17(9): 595–604.

Maslow JN, Mulligan ME, Arbeit RD (1993) Molecular epidemiology: application of contemporary techniques to the typing of microorganisms. Clinical Infectious Disease 17(2): 153–62; quiz 163–4. [Comment: Clinical Infectious Disease (1994) 18(6): 1017–19.]

May RM, Anderson RM (1987) Transmission dynamics of HIV infection. Nature 326(6109): 137–42.

Mays N, Pope C (1995) Qualitative research: Observational methods in health care settings. British Medical Journal 311(6998): 182–4.

McFarland LV (1993) Diarrhea acquired in the hospital. Gastroenterology Clinics of North America 22(3): 563–77.

McFarland LV, Mulligan ME, Kwok RY, Stamm WE (1989) Nosocomial acquisition of Clostridium difficile infection. New England Journal of Medicine 320(4): 204–10. [Comment: New England Journal of Medicine (1989) 321(3): 190.]

McGinnis MR, Sigler L, Rinaldi MG (1999) Some medically important fungi and their common synonyms and names of uncertain application. Clinical Infectious Diseases 29(4): 728–30.

Meers PD, Yeo GA (1978) Shedding of bacteria and skin squames after handwashing. Journal of Hygiene (London) 81(1): 99–105.

Mermel LA, Farr BM, Sherertz RJ, Raad II, O'Grady N, Harris JS, Craven DE; Infectious Diseases Society of America, American College of Critical Care Medicine, Society for Healthcare Epidemiology of America (2001a) Guidelines for the management of intravascular catheter-related infections. Clinical Infectious Disease 32(9): 1249–72.

Mermel LA, Farr BM, Sherertz RJ, Raad II, O'Grady N, Harris JS, Craven DE (2001b) Guidelines for the management of intravascular catheter-related infections. Infection Control and Hospital Epidemiology 22(4): 222–42.

Mertens R, Kegels G, Stroobant A, Reybrouck G, Lamotte JM, Potvliege C, Van Casteren V, Lauwers S, Verschraegen G, Wauters G, et al. (1987) The national prevalence survey of nosocomial infections in Belgium, 1984. Journal of Hospital Infection 9(3): 219–29.

Miller MJ (1999a) A Guide to Specimen Management in Clinical Microbiology, 2nd edn. Washington DC, ASM Press.

Miller MJ (1999b) Viral taxonomy. Clinical Infectious Diseases 29(4): 731–33.

Mims CA, Nash A, Stephen J (2001) Mims' Pathogenesis of Infectious Diseases, 5th edn. San Diego: Academic Press.

Mollison D (Ed) (1995) Epidemic Models: Their Structure and Relation to Data. Cambridge: Cambridge University Press.

Moro ML, Stazi MA, Marasca G, Greco D, Zampieri (1986) A National prevalence survey of hospital-acquired infections in Italy, 1983. Journal of Hospital Infection 8(1): 72–85.

Morris T, Brecher SM, Fitzsimmons D, Durbin A, Arbeit RD, Maslow JN (1995) A pseudoepidemic due to laboratory contamination deciphered by molecular analysis. Infection Control and Hospital Epidemiology 16(2): 82–7.

Muench H (1959) Catalytic Models in Epidemiology. Cambridge, Mass: Harvard University Press.

Nickel JC, Gristina AG, Costerton JW (1985) Electron microscopic study of an infected Foley catheter. Canadian Journal of Surgery 28(1): 50–1.

O'Connor HJ, Axon AT (1983) Gastrointestinal endoscopy: infection and disinfection. Gut 24(11): 1067–77.

Oliveira D, Santos-Sanches I, Mato R, Tamayo M, Ribeiro G, Costa D, de Lencastre H (1998) Virtually all methicillin-resistant Staphylococcus aureus (MRSA) infections in the largest Portuguese teaching hospital are caused by two internationally spread multiresistant strains: the Iberian and the Brazilian clones of MRSA. Clinical Microbiology and Infection 4(7): 373–85.

Olson MM, Lee JT Jr (1990) Continuous, 10-year wound infection surveillance: results, advantages, and unanswered questions. Archives of Surgery 125(6): 794–803.

Owens WD, Felts JA, Spitznagel EL Jr (1978) ASA physical status classifications: a study of consistency of ratings. Anesthesiology 49(4): 239–43.

Pearson ML, Hospital Infection Control Practices Advisory Committee (1996a) Guideline for prevention of intravascular device-related infections. Infection Control and Hospital Epidemiology 17(7): 438–73. [Comment: Infection Control Hospital Epidemiology (1998) 19(10): 739.]

Pearson ML, The Hospital Infection Control Practices Advisory Committee (1996b) Guideline for prevention of intravascular device-related infections, Part I: Intravascular device-related infections: an overview. American Journal of Infection Control 24(4): 262–77.

Pierce AK, Sanford JP, Thomas GD, Leonard JS (1970) Long-term evaluation of decontamination of inhalation-therapy equipment and the occurrence of necrotizing pneumonia. New England Journal of Medicine 282(10): 528–31.

Pope C, Mays N (1995) Reaching the parts other methods cannot reach: an introduction to qualitative methods in health and health services research. British Medical Journal 311(6996): 42–45. [Comment: British Medical Journal (1995) 311(6996): 2.]

Quade D, Culver DH, Haley RW, Whaley FS, Kalsbeek WD, Hardison CD, Johnson RE, Stanley RC, Shachtman RH (1980a) The SENIC sampling process: design for choosing hospitals and patients and results of sample selection. American Journal of Epidemiology 111(5): 486–502.

Quade D, Lachenbruch PA, Whaley FS, McClish DK, Haley RW (1980b) Effects of misclassifications on statistical inferences in epidemiology. American Journal of Epidemiology 111(5): 503–15.

Raahave D, Friis-Moller A, Bjerre-Jepsen K, Thiis-Knudsen J, Rasmussen LB (1986) The infective dose of aerobic and anaerobic bacteria in postoperative wound sepsis. Archives of Surgery 121(8): 924–9.

Rammelkamp CH, Mortimer EA, Wolinsky E (1964) Transmission of Streptococcal and Staphylococcal infections. Annals of Internal Medicine 60: 753–8.

Rodrigues LC, Diwan VD, Wheeler JG (1993) Protective effect of BCG against tuberculosis meningitis and military tuberculosis: a meta analysis. International Journal of Epidemiology 22(6): 1154–8.

Rodrigues LC, Noel Gill O, Smith PG (1991) BCG vaccination in the first year of life protects children of Indian subcontinent ethnic origin against tuberculosis in England. Journal of Epidemiology and Community Health 45(1): 78–80.

Rothman KJ (1976) Causes. American Journal of Epidemiology 104(6): 587–92.

Rowan KM, Kerr JH, Major E, McPherson K, Short A, Vessey MP (1993a) Intensive Care Society's APACHE II study in Britain and Ireland, I: Variations in case mix of adult admissions to general intensive care units and impact on outcome. British Medical Journal 307(6910): 972–7. [Comment: British Medical Journal (1993) 307(6910): 953–4.]

Rowan KM, Kerr JH, Major E, McPherson K, Short A, Vessey MP (1993b) Intensive Care Society's APACHE II study in Britain and Ireland, II: Outcome comparisons of intensive care units after adjustment for case mix by the American APACHE II method. British Medical Journal 307(6910): 977–81. [Comment: British Medical Journal (1993) 307(6910): 953–4.]

Saklad M (1941) Grading of patients for surgical procedures. Anesthesiology 2: 281–4.

Sanders CV Jr, Luby JP, Johanson WG Jr, Barnett JA, Sanford JP (1970) Serratia marcescens infections from inhalation therapy medications: nosocomial outbreak. Annals of Internal Medicine 73(1): 15–21.

Saviteer SM, Samsa GP, Rutala WA (1988) Nosocomial infections in the elderly. Increased risk per hospital day. American Journal of Medicine 84(4): 661–6.

Semmelweis Ignaz Philip (1861) Etiologie und Prophylaxis des Kindbettfiebers [The Aetiology, the Concept and the Prophylaxis of Childbed Fever]. Pest: Hartleben.

Seropian R, Reynolds BM (1971) Wound infections after preoperative depilatory versus razor preparation. American Journal of Surgery 121(3): 251–4.

Stamm WE (1975) Guidelines for prevention of catheter-associated urinary tract infections. Annals of Internal Medicine 82(3): 386–90.

Stamm WE, Hooton TM, Johnson JR, Johnson C, Stapleton A, Roberts PL, Moseley SL, Fihn SD (1989) Urinary tract infections: from pathogenesis to treatment. Journal of Infectious Disease 159(3): 400–6.

Stamm WE, Hooton TM (1993) Management of urinary tract infections in adults. New England Journal of Medicine 329(18): 1328–34. [Comment: New England Journal of Medicine (1994) 330(11): 792; New England Journal of Medicine (1994) 331(9): 617–18.]

Stamm WE, Weinstein RA, Dixon RE (1981) Comparison of endemic and epidemic nosocomial infections. American Journal of Medicine 70(2): 393–7.

Stark RP, Maki DG (1984) Bacteriuria in the catheterized patient. What quantitative level of bacteriuria is relevant? New England Journal of Medicine 311(9): 560–4.

Tablan OC, Anderson LJ, Arden NH, Breiman RF, Butler JC, McNeil MM, The Hospital Infection Control Practices Advisory Committee, Centers for Disease Control and Prevention (1994a) Guideline for prevention of nosocomial pneumonia. Infection Control and Hospital Epidemiology 15(9): 587–627. [Erratum: Infection Control and Hospital Epidemiology (1998) 19(5): 304.]

Tablan OC, Anderson LJ, Arden NH, Breiman RF, Butler JC, McNeil MM, The Hospital Infection Control Practices Advisory Committee, Centers for Disease Control and Prevention (1994b) Guideline for prevention of nosocomial pneumonia. American Journal of Infection Control 22(4): 247–92. [Erratum: American Journal of Infection Control (1994b) 22(6): 351; American Journal of Infection Control (1994) 22(5): 324.]

Taylor LJ (1978a) An evaluation of handwashing techniques, 1. Nursing Times 74(2): 54–55.

Taylor LJ (1978b) An evaluation of handwashing techniques, 2. Nursing Times 74(3): 108–10.

Teasdale G, Jennett B (1974) Assessment of coma and impaired consciousness. A practical scale. Lancet 2(7872): 81–4.

Teasdale G, Murray G, Parker L, Jennett B (1979) Adding up the Glasgow Coma Score. Acta Neurochirurgica Suppl (Wien); 28(1): 13–6.

Tess BH, Glenister HM, Rodrigues LC, Wagner MB (1993) Incidence of hospital-acquired infection and length of hospital stay. European Journal of Clinical Microbiology and Infectious Disease 12(2): 81–6.

Thacker SB, Berkelman RL (1988) Public health surveillance in the United States. Epidemiologic Reviews 10: 164–90.

Thacker SB, Parrish RG, Trowbridge F (1988) A method for evaluating systems of epidemiological surveillance World Health Statistics Quarterly 41(1): 11–18. [Erratum: World Health Statistics Quarterly (1989) 42(2): preceding 58.]

Thoburn R, Fekety FR Jr, Cluff LE, Melvin VB (1968) Infections acquired by hospitalized patients. An analysis of the overall problem. Archives of Internal Medicine 121(1): 1–10.

Top FH (Ed) (1967) Control of Infectious Diseases in General Hospitals. New York: American Public Health Association.

United States Department of Health and Human Services (1992) Principles of Epidemiology: An Introduction to Applied Epidemiology and Biostatistics. Atlanta, Ga: USDHHS.

United States Pharmacopeial Convention (2000) The United States Pharmacopoeia, 24th edn. Rockville, MD: United States Pharmacopeial Convention.

Vogt RL, LaRue D, Klaucke DN, Jillson DA (1983) Comparison of an active and passive surveillance system of primary care providers for hepatitis, measles, rubella, and salmonellosis in Vermont. American Journal of Public Health 73(7): 795–7.

Weinstein RA, Stamm WE (1977) Pseudoepidemics in hospital. Lancet 2(8043): 862–4.

Wenzel RP, Reagan DR, Bertino JS Jr, Baron EJ, Arias K (1998) Methicillin-resistant Staphylococcus aureus outbreak: a consensus panel's definition and management guidelines. American Journal of Infection Control 26(2): 102–10.

Whaley FS, Quade D, Haley RW (1980) Effects of method error on the power of a statistical test. Implications of imperfect sensitivity and specificity in retrospective chart review. American Journal of Epidemiology 111(5): 534–42.

Wharton M, Chorba TL, Vogt RL, Morse DL, Buehler JW (1990) Case definitions for public health surveillance. Morbidity and Mortality Weekly Report 39(RR-13): 1–43.

Williams RE (1966) Epidemiology of airborne staphylococcal infection. Bacteriology Reviews 30(3): 660–74.

Wilson FA (1995) Understanding Digital Technology. London: Bernard Babani.

Working Party (1998) Report: Received guidelines for the control of methicillin-resistant Staphylococcus aureus infection in hospitals. Journal of Hospital Infection 39: 253–90.

World Health Organization (1996) Immunization Policy. Global Programme for Vaccines and Immunization. Expanded Programme on Immunization. Geneva: WHO.

World Health Organization (1999) Infection Control Guidelines for Transmissible Spongiform Encephalopathies: Report of a WHO Consultation, 23–26 March. WHO/CDS/CSR/APH/2000.3. Geneva: WHO.

Zhang YX (1987) A compound catalytic model with both reversible and two-stage types and its applications in epidemiological study. International Journal of Epidemiology 16(4): 619–21.

Bibliography

Advisory Committee on Immunization Practices. American Academy of Pediatrics. American Academy of Family Physicians. National Immunization Program, CDC (1995) Recommended childhood immunization schedule – United States, January 1995. Morbidity and Mortality Weekly Report 43(51–52): 959–60. [Erratum: Morbidity and Mortality Weekly Report (1995) 44(9): 174–5.]

American Society for Healthcare Central Service Personnel of the American Hospital Association (1989) Recommended Practice for Central Service, Section Six: Sterilization.

Association of Operating Room Nurses (AORN) (2000) Standards, Recommended Practices and Guidelines. Revised. AORN: 347–58.

Benett JV, Brachman PS (Eds) (1998) Nosocomial Infections, 4th edn. Philadelphia: Lippincott-Raven.

Block SS (Ed) (2000) Disinfection, Sterilization, and Preservation, 5th edn. Philadelphia: Lippincott Williams & Wilkins.

Garner JS, Favero MS (1985) CDC Guideline for Handwashing and Hospital Environmental Control. Infection Control 7(4): 231–43.

Garner JS, Favero MS (1985) CDC guidelines for the prevention and control of nosocomial infections. Guideline for handwashing and hospital environmental control. Supersedes guideline for hospital environmental control published in 1981. American Journal of Infection Control 14(3): 110–29.

Garner JS, Hughes JM, (1987) Options for isolation precautions. Annals of Internal Medicine 107(2): 248–50.

Mandell GL, Bennett JE, Dolin R (Eds) (1995) Principles and Practice of Infectious Diseases, 4th edn. New York: Churchill Livingstone.

McCulloch J (Ed) (2000) Infection Control. Science, Management and Practice. London and Philadelphia: Whurr Publishers.

Murray PR, Baron EJ, Pfaller MA, Tenover FC, Yolken RH (Eds) (1995) Manual of Clinical Microbiology, 6th edn. Washington: ASM Press.

Annexe 1

American National Standards in United States regulating sterilization in hospitals and in industry

Issuer, number and year of publication	Title
ANSI/AAMI ST8:1994	Hospital steam sterilizers 3rd edn
ANSI/AAMI ST19:1999	Biological indicators – Part 3: Biological indicators for moist heat sterilization, 2nd edn
ANSI/AAMI ST21:1999	Biological indicators – Part 2: Biological indicators for EO sterilization, 2nd edn
ANSI/AAMI ST24:1999	Automatic, general-purpose EO sterilizers and EO sterilant sources intended for use in health care facilities, 3rd edn
ANSI/AAMI ST33:1996	Guidelines for the selection and use of reusable rigid container systems for ethylene oxide sterilization and steam sterilization in health care facilities, 2nd edn
ANSI/AAMI ST34:1991	Guideline for the use of ethylene oxide and steam biological indicators in industrial sterilization processes, 1st edn
ANSI/AAMI ST35:1996	Safe handling and biological decontamination of medical devices in health care facilities and non-medical settings, 2nd edn
ANSI/AAMI ST37:1996	Flash sterilization – Steam sterilization of patient care items for immediate use, 3rd edn
ANSI/AAMI ST40:1992/(R)1998	Table-top dry heat (heated air) sterilization and sterility assurance in dental and medical facilities, 1st edn
ANSI/AAMI ST41:1999	Ethylene oxide sterilization in health care facilities: Safety and effectiveness, 3rd edn
ANSI/AAMI ST42:1998	Steam sterilization and sterility assurance using table-top sterilizers in office-based, ambulatory-care, medical, surgical and dental facilities, 2nd edn
ANSI/AAMI ST44:1992	BIER/EO gas vessels, 2nd edn, errata issued 1994
ANSI/AAMI ST45:1992	BIER/steam vessels, 2nd edn
ANSI/AAMI ST46:1993	Good hospital practice: Steam sterilization and sterility assurance, 3rd edn
ANSI/AAMI ST50:1995	Dry heat (heated air) sterilizers, 1st edn

ANSI/AAMI ST55:1997	Table-top sterilizers, 1st edn
ANSI/AAMI ST58:1996	Safe use and handling of glutaraldehyde-based products in health care facilities, 1st edn
ANSI/AAMI ST59:1999	Sterilization of health care products – Biological indicators-Part 1: General, 1st edn
ANSI/AAMI ST60:1996	Sterilization of health care products – Chemical indicators-Part 1: General requirements, 1st edn
ANSI/AAMI ST66:1999	Sterilization of health care products – Chemical indicators-Part 2: Class 2 indicators for air removal test, 1st edn
ANSI/AAMI/ISO 11134:1993	Requirements for validation and routine control – Industrial moist heat sterilization, 2nd edn
ANSI/AAMI/ISO 11135:1994	Medical devices – Validation and routine control of ethylene oxide sterilization, 3rd edn, errata issued 1995
ANSI/AAMI/ISO 11137:1994	Requirements for validation and routine control – Radiation sterilization 3rd edn, errata issued 1997
ANSI/AAMI/ISO 11607:1997	Packaging for terminally sterilized medical devices, 1st edn
ANSI/AAMI/ISO 11737-1:1995	Microbiological methods – Part 1: Estimation of the population of micro-organisms on product, 1st edn
AAMI/ISO 117-2:1998	Microbiological methods – Part 2: Test of sterility performed in the validation of sterilization process, 1st edn
AAMI/ISO 14160:1998	Sterilization of single-use medical devices incorporating materials of animal origin – Validation and routine control of sterilization by liquid chemical sterilants, 1st edn
AAMI TIR7:1990	Chemical sterilants and high level disinfectants: A guide to selection and use, 2nd edn
AAMI TIR12:1994	Designing, testing and labelling reusable medical devices for reprocessing in health care facilities: A guide for device manufacturers, 1st edn
AAMI TIR13:1997	Principles of industrial moist heat sterilization, 1st edn
AAMI TIR14:1997	Contract sterilization for ethylene oxide, 1st edn
AAMI TIR15:1997	Ethylene oxide sterilization equipment, process considerations and pertinent calculations, 1st edn
AAMI TIR17:1997	Radiation sterilization – Material qualification, 1st edn

AAMI TIR19:1998 and TIR19/A:1999	Guidance for ANSI/AAMI/ISO 10993-7: 1995, Biological evaluation of medical devices – Part 7: Ethylene oxide sterilization residuals, 1st edn and Amendment
AAMI TIR22:1998	Guidance for ANSI/AAMI/ISO 11607: 1997, Packaging for terminally sterilized medical devices, 1st edn
AAMI TIR25:1999	Chemical indicators – Guidance for the selection, use, and interpretation of results in health care facilities, 2nd edn
AAMI/ISO TIR 13409:1996	Radiation sterilization – Substantiation of 25 kGy as a sterilization dose for small or infrequent production batches, 1st edn
AAMI/ISO TIR 15844:1998	Radiation sterilization – Selection of a sterilization dose for a single production batch, 1st edn

ANSI = American National Standards Institute; AAMI = Association for the Advancement of Medical Instrumentation; ISO = International Organization for Standardization; TIR = Technical Information Report.

Annexe 2

Standards of the European Union regulating sterilization in hospitals

Issuer	Number	Title	Accepted
CEN	EN 285	Sterilization – Steam sterilizers – Large sterilizers	08 Nov. 1997
CEN	EN 455-1	Medical gloves for single use – Part 1: Requirements and testing for absence of holes	18 Nov. 1995
CEN	EN 455-2	Medical gloves for single use – Part 2: Requirements and testing for physiological properties	18 Nov. 1995
CEN	EN 475	Medical devices. Electrically generated alarm signals	18 Nov. 1995
CEN	EN 540	Clinical investigation of medical devices for humans	18. Nov. 1995
CEN	EN 550	Sterilization of medical devices – Validation and routine control of ethylene oxide sterilization	04 Oct. 1994
CEN	EN 552	Sterilization of medical devices – Validation and routine control of sterilization by irradiation	04 Oct. 1994
CEN	EN 554	Sterilization of medical devices – Validation and routine control of by moist heat	04 Oct. 1994
CEN	EN 556	Sterilization of medical devices – Requirements for medical devices to be labelled 'Sterile'	18 Nov. 1995
CEN	EN 724	Guidance on the application of EN 29001 and EN 46001 and of EN 29002 and 46002 for non-active medical devices	18 Nov. 1995
CEN	EN 867-2	Non-biological systems for use in sterilizers – Part 2: Process indicators (Class A)	08 Nov. 1997
CEN	EN 867-3	Non-biological systems for use in sterilizers – Part 3: Specification for Class B indicators for use in the Bowie and Dick test	08 Nov. 1997
CEN	EN 868-1	Packing materials and systems for medical devices which are to be sterilized – Part 1: General requirements and test methods.	17 May 1997
CEN	EN 1174-1	Sterilization of medical devices – Estimation of the population of micro-organisms on product – Part 1: Requirements	23 Aug. 1996
CEN	EN 1174-2	Sterilization of medical devices – Estimation of the population of micro-organisms on product – Part 2: Guidance	17 May 1997

CEN	EN 1174-3	Sterilization of medical devices – Estimation of the population of micro-organisms on product – Part 3: Guide to the methods for validation of microbiological techniques	17 May 1997
CEN	EN 1422	Sterilizers for medical purposes – Ethylene oxide sterilizers – Requirements and test method	09 May 1998
CEN	EN ISO 10993-10	Sterile, single-use intravascular catheters – Part 1: General requirements (ISO 10555-1:1995)	17 May 1997
CEN	EN ISO 10993-10	Biological evaluation of medical devices – Part 10: tests for irritation and sensitization (ISO 10993-10: 1995)	17 May 1997
CEN	EN ISO 10993-12	Biological evaluation of medical devices – Part 12: Sample preparation and reference materials (ISO 10993-12:1996)	19 May 1997

CEN = Comité Européen de Normalisation (European Commitee for Standardization).

Annexe 3

Required amount of disinfectant for an appropriate concentration of total solution in the SI system

	Concentration of the required solution							
	0.25%	0.5%	1%	2%	3%	4%	5%	10%
Total amount of the solution in litres (l)	Amount of the disinfectant ingredient in grams (g) for the appropriate solution							
1	2.5	5	10	20	30	40	50	100
2	5	10	20	40	60	80	100	200
3	7.5	15	30	60	90	120	150	300
4	10	20	40	80	120	160	200	400
5	12.5	25	50	100	150	200	250	500
6	15	30	60	120	180	240	300	600
7	17.5	35	70	140	210	280	350	700
8	20	40	80	160	240	320	400	800
9	22.5	45	90	180	270	360	450	900
10	25	50	100	200	300	400	500	1000
15	37.5	75	150	300	450	600	750	1500
20	50	100	200	400	600	800	1000	2000
30	75	150	300	600	900	1200	1500	3000
50	125	250	500	1000	1500	2000	2500	5000

If the viscosity of the disinfectant is equal to one gram per ml then the amount of the disinfectant will be the same in ml as in grams.

Index